fusion fitness

15 MARTIAL ART WORKOUTS FOR MIND, BODY AND SPIRIT

on my way
August 6·08
290 lbs

D1410356

fusion fitness

15 MARTIAL ART WORKOUTS FOR MIND, BODY AND SPIRIT

anne-marie millard

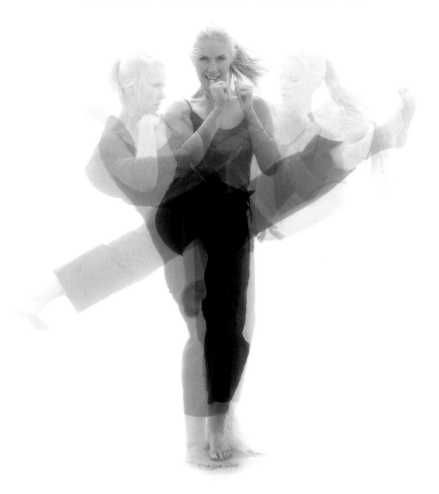

KYLE CATHIE LIMITED

TO
Kenneth E. Millard and Emilie Koreska Millard

My combined oracles of all
truth and knowledge

First published in Great Britain 2003 by
Kyle Cathie Limited
122 Arlington Road
London NW1 7HP
general.enquiries@kyle-cathie.com
www.kylecathie.com

ISBN 1 85626 462 9

Text © 2003 Anne-Marie Millard
Design and layout © Kyle Cathie Limited 2003
Special photography © Tim Winter

Senior Editor: Helen Woodhall
Editorial Assistant: Esme West
Designer: Mark Buckingham
Production: Sha Huxtable and Lorraine Baird
Index: Helen Snaith
Hair and makeup: Emily Cooper

Anne-Marie Millard is hereby identified as the author of this work
in accordance with Section 77 of the Copyright, Designs and Patents Act 1988.

A Cataloguing In Publication record for this title is available from the British Library.

Colour separations by Scanhouse Ltd.
Printed in Singapore by Kyodo Printing Co.

INTRODUCTION

Millions of people world-wide practise martial arts. Through their various disciplines these men, women and children are learning how to improve their fitness, health, self-awareness, confidence and self-defence levels. Many people are put off martial arts because of the popular misconception that they begin and end with violence. However anyone who has even begun to learn a martial art from a reputable teacher knows that nothing is further from the truth. The guiding principles of courtesy, respect and self-discipline are inherent in all martial arts teaching. Rather than fighting other people, a good martial artist should know the benefit of first fighting the enemy within. The manifold rewards both of making an effort to become a better person and of the inner strengths that can be gained from martial arts training can greatly increase one's quality of life.

Another problem seems to be the overwhelming amount of differing systems within the arts. You might be interested in learning – but where do you start? tai chi or tae kwon do? What is the difference? How do the benefits vary? Faced with such questions and with little available information, the consensus seems to be to avoid the whole lot.

The purpose of this book is two-fold. First, to help you improve your health and fitness levels in a simple and effective way. Second, to increase your knowledge of the martial arts and to inspire you to delve deeper into its world. It is very difficult, if not impossible, to teach yourself a martial art properly; instruction in person by an experienced, insured, qualified and professionally recognised person is essential. However I have endeavoured to bring you a taster of some of the more widely taught martial arts.

The workouts within this book have been devised from several different martial art styles, some of which are inter-related (more on that later), and they each have certain benefits. For example, Tae Kwon Do is well known for its dynamic kicks, so I have taken some simple moves from this powerful kicking martial art and developed them into a high-energy workout.

The philosophy behind this book is simple. In our quest for health and fitness we all need to find an activity that we enjoy. Too many people become slave to the treadmill and then wonder why they lose interest after six weeks. Our bodies abide by the laws of nature – it is our conscious mind that does not. We have stopped listening to our bodies and consistently fight against the natural order. Our energy levels, moods and feelings fluctuate daily, so to follow a rigid regime of one exercise is ineffective and unnecessary. A shifting programme of exercise that you can dip in and out of not only gives you a greater variety but ultimately gives you a much improved level of fitness. The workouts are like a simple puzzle: however you choose to put the pieces together, the outcome is the same. I hope you enjoy this book and that it gives you all the fitness and fulfilment that martial arts have given me.

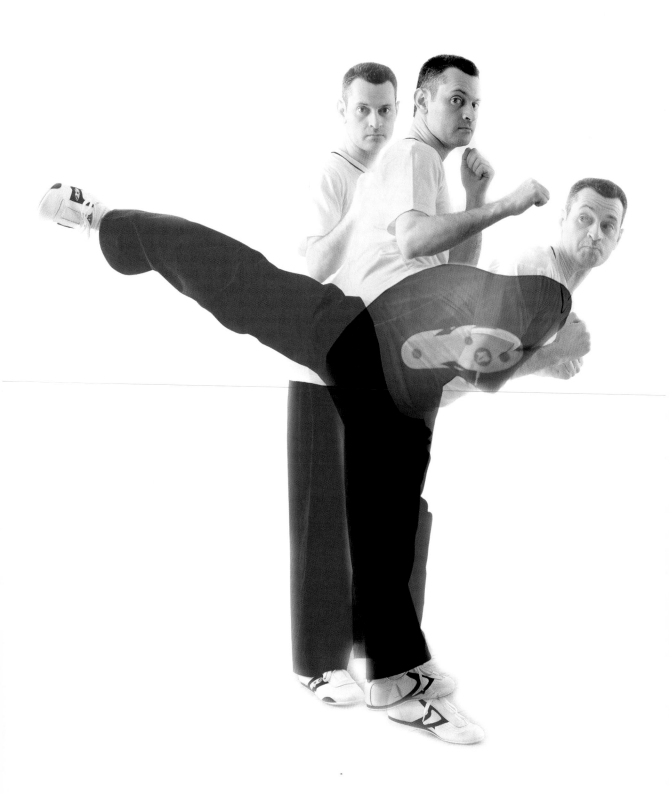

Over the centuries martial arts have proliferated. Various teachers have developed certain techniques and changed emphasis, and then given names to their 'new' methods.

WHAT ARE MARTIAL ARTS? >>

Like branches of a tree or a very enthusiastic grapevine, different styles of martial arts continue to ramify into even more complex schools and ways of thought. It would be impossible for this book to even begin to touch on all the styles. Therefore I have tried to give you a brief overview of a few of those that are more widely available.

WING CHUN

Like aikido, Wing Chun kuen kung fu is a relative newcomer to the world of martial arts. It is attributed to a woman called Yin Wing Chun, who was a protégé of a Buddhist nun called Ng Mui. Wing Chun is known as a 'soft' style, but is in fact a blend of 'hard' and 'soft' techniques.

Whereas a hard style is involves meeting force with force, a soft style is one that uses more evasive manoeuvres and techniques.

Roughly translated, 'wing chun' means 'beautiful springtime' and 'kuen' means 'fist' or 'fist fighting style'. However the majority of the time, this martial art is referred to as simply 'wing chun'. This blending of hard and soft styles is due to the fact that it was developed by a woman and refined mainly by men. It is centred on the Taoist principle of 'take the middle road'. In essence, this says that you should not go to extremes, and that success is based on balance. If you are on the middle road you can see both the left and right paths, but if you venture too much to one side you may lose sight of the other. This can also be interpreted as the concept of the hard and soft principles – or yin and yang. Yin (the feminine side) focuses on diverting the flow of energy; Yang (the masculine side) seeks to resist any opposing energy flow.

This style, originally favoured by Bruce Lee before he created jeet kune do, features a characteristic turned-in style with the body facing forwards and the hands protecting the centre line; the opponent is attacked from close quarters. It is also well-known for its 'sticky hands' (chi sau) technique. To the uninitiated, this technique is best described as a hurt boxer trying to 'spoil' his opponent's moves by clinging to his arms. The aim is to prevent an opponent from striking freely, giving the wing chun practitioner the opportunity to control, trap and break free to strike. The real skill lies in both parties wanting to achieve the same goal, and this has led to exceptional techniques, in which either one or both parties can train blindfold.

TAI CHI CHUAN >>

This martial art is said to have been created by the Taoist immortal Chang San-feng, a twelfth-century recluse who lived in the Wu-tang mountains, in Hupeh Province. He witnessed a fight between a snake and a crane, in which the crane's stabbing attack was neutralised by the snake's twisting movements. He saw in this struggle living proof of the Taoist belief stated in the *Tao Te Ching* by the ancient master, Lao Tzu: 'The most yielding of things in the universe overcomes the most hard' (v. 43). Inspired by this, he created tai chi chuan.

Unfortunately, this story is almost certainly untrue. The style seems to have originated in Chen village, Hunan Province. It passed to Yang Lu-chan who founded the Yang style. There are other styles, including the Chen village style, the Sun style (founded by Sun Lu-t'ang, 1859–1933) and the Wu (founded by Wu Chien Chuan, 1870–1942) as well as a modern style, developed on the mainland.

Tai chi chuan works on a number of levels, but its principal aim is to teach practitioners to relax and become fluid in their movements. This leads to smoother actions and quicker response times. It is also known as 'internal kung fu', as it emphasises the development of the internal aspects of the body – breathing, flexibility and the mind – as opposed to external tension or muscular strength. The term 'tai chi chuan' is usually translated as 'the supreme ultimate fist'. 'Tai chi' refers to the Chinese yin-yang symbol, also known as the hard and soft sign – symbolising two opposites coming together. 'Chuan' refers to a boxing method – a method of empty-hand combat, in this context, rather than a sporting contest.

Tai chi chuan training includes punches, kicks, locks, open-hand techniques and throws in its repertoire, as well as traditional Chinese weapons: sword, broadsword, staff and spear. It incorporates chi kung exercises, which encourage deep breathing, improved blood circulation and greater efficiency of all the body's systems. The calm concentration required for its practice can bring about a serene state of mind that is useful in helping to eradicate daily stresses and strains.

This martial art is open to anyone. Age, health or infirmity is no barrier to beginning to practise tai chi and chi kung, although it does require more demanding practice to reach some of the higher levels.

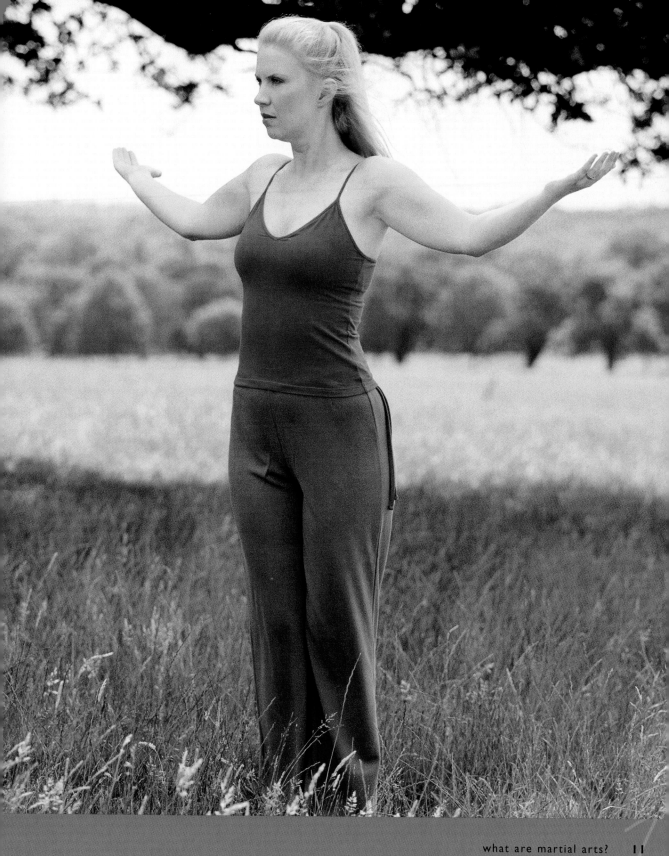

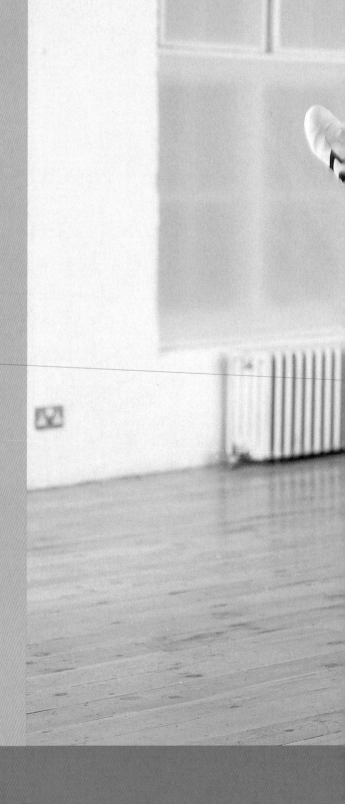

KICKBOXING   >>

Kickboxing is a relatively modern martial arts system. It combines fighting techniques from more traditional systems, such as Kyokushinkai karate, kung fu, Thai boxing, tae kwon do and kyokky shinkai. It does not contain a lot of fancy footwork; nor does it have long-standing philosophies and creeds. Instead, it offers no-frills fighting that focuses on power, strength, flexibility, stamina and a blatant urge to win.

Martial arts boomed during the early 1970s and interest was greatly increased by an emphasis on competition fighting. Chinese styles of fighting began to be Westernised in the UK, and even more so in the United States, where the first real freestyle systems were being created. Many traditional martial artists, frustrated with the limitations of competition scoring, wished to see how effective their moves would be in a more realistic environment. They focused on specialised techniques, such as kicks and punches, being delivered with full-force.

Today, fights and tournaments are staged all over the Western world and many modern fitness hybrids, such as cardio kickboxing and tae bo, have originated from it.

THAI BOXING (MUAY THAI)

This is considered to be one of the most devastating fighting systems in the world. It uses the full range of natural weapons to defeat an opponent. The modern version has been influenced by Western boxing, improving the punching and defensive skills of the fighters, but the knee, elbow and shin techniques are derived from the traditional art. It is a fast-moving and dynamic martial art which teaches speed, power, mental agility and increases stamina.

In the past muay Thai was practised by warriors as part of their martial training. According to tradition, Yi Kumkam became king of Thailand by defeating his brother Fang Ken in a boxing match. This method avoided the bloodshed of a civil war which could have destroyed the country.

Thai boxers are considered to be skilled in the use of the leg, knee and elbow. Grappling is not permitted and there is no ground fighting. Muay Thai is open to both men and women.

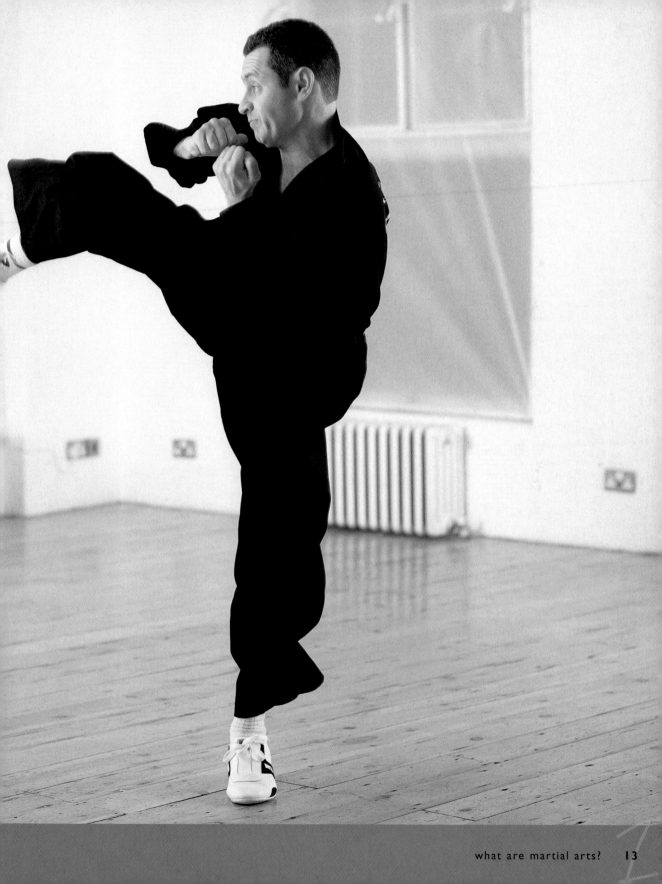

KARATE 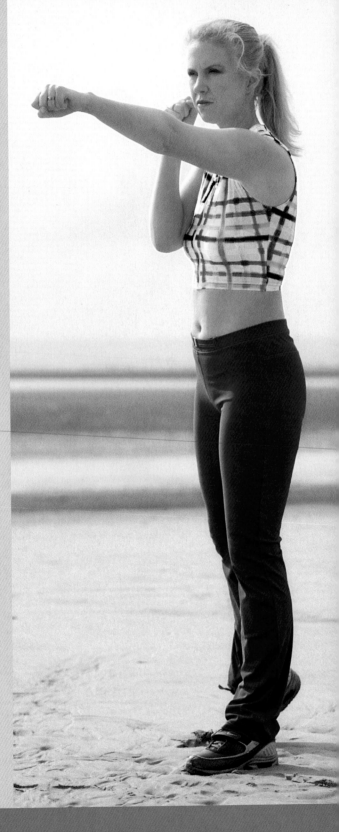 >>

Karate, or karate-do, simply translated means 'empty hand' ('kara' means 'empty' and 'te' means 'hand'), and this martial art is predominantly concerned with fighting with bare hands and feet. The basic principle is to turn the body into an effective weapon to defend and attack.

Karate is one of the most widely practised of the oriental martial arts. It evolved during one of the Japanese occupations of the island of Okinawa, part of the Ryukyu chain of islands, in the fifteenth century. Its roots, however, can be traced much further back – all the way to ancient India and China. Many people believe that the 'oriental' martial arts have their roots in India. Indeed, when we look at such disciplines such as yoga, there do seem to be certain similarities.

It is believed that Zen Buddhist monks took the Indian fighting techniques to China as early as the fifth and sixth centuries BC. Bodidharmi, the most famous of these monks, travelled at the end of the fifth century AD from India to China, where he became an instructor at the Shaolin monastery. He taught a combination of empty hand fighting systems and yoga, and this became known as Shaolin kung fu – the system on which many Chinese martial arts systems are based.

In 1470, the Japanese had occupied the island of Okinawa and decreed that anybody found carrying weapons would be put to death. To protect themselves from local bandits, who by and large ignored the prohibition on weapons, Zen Buddhist monks developed the empty-hand system known as te ('hand'), importing new techniques from China. Eventually the new art was translated as t'ang ('China hand'), but was familiarly known as Okinawa-te ('Okinawa hand'). In the twentieth century t'ang became known as karate-do ('empty hand').

There are numerous styles of karate and the The Mind Maze workout in chapter six features a style called goju ryu. It is said to display the oldest martial art traditions, with a history that can be traced back 2000 years. It reflects the primitive traditional forms of martial arts yet is full of fighting spirit. The system is based on a concept that hard and stiff is not good, but that all soft and gentle can be equally harmful. The two should complement each other. This combination of the two gives goju ryu its beauty, disciplined moves, grace and flowing form.

AIKIDO

Created by Morihei Ueshiba (1883–1969), aikido in its present form is a relatively recent innovation within the martial arts tradition. Ueshiba was introduced to the classical martial arts as a boy by his father, Yoroku. He is known to have studied some martial arts, such as various styles of ju jitsu as well as kenjutsu and the art of the spear. In 1912 Morihei moved to Hokkaido, where a chance meeting with a man called Sokaku Takeda changed his life.

Takeda was a master of daito ryu-aiki ju jitsu, a martial art that originated in the sixth century AD and had been passed down through the military hierarchy and formalised by members of the Aizu clan, becoming known as oshikiuchi, or 'striking arts'. The young Ueshibi studied under Takeda until 1919. Then, on returning to his native Tanabe on the death of his father, Morihei met Onisaburo Deguchi, the charismatic founder of an esoteric religion called Omoto-Kyo, and spent the next six years as his disciple, travelling throughout Asia.

In 1927, Morihei set up the Kobukan dojo in Tokyo and began teaching an amalgam of the martial traditions he had learnt from Takeda, together with the spiritual beliefs he had gleaned from Deguchi. This new discipline, firstly known as Ueshiba aiko-budo, became finally known as aikido. This word is a combination of three concepts: 'ai' meaning 'harmony'; 'ki' meaning 'spirit'; and 'do' meaning 'way'. In a spiritual sense, this means harmonising your individual spirit, or ki, with the spirit of nature itself. In the dojo, this means that you harmonise with an attack, lead it to a point of exhaustion and then neutralise it with a throw, a joint lock, or an immobilisation.

Aikido is a discipline that seeks not to meet violence with violence, but instead looks towards harmonising with and restraining an opponent. Often recognised by the distinctive hakama (a divided or pleated black skirt) which students are entitled to wear after passing their first dan (black belt) exam, aikido training incorporates knife taking, sword and stick taking, and even defence from a kneeling position.

It is a martial art that can be learned for a variety of reasons: as a way of becoming physically fit, as self-defence; or to understand something of Japanese culture.

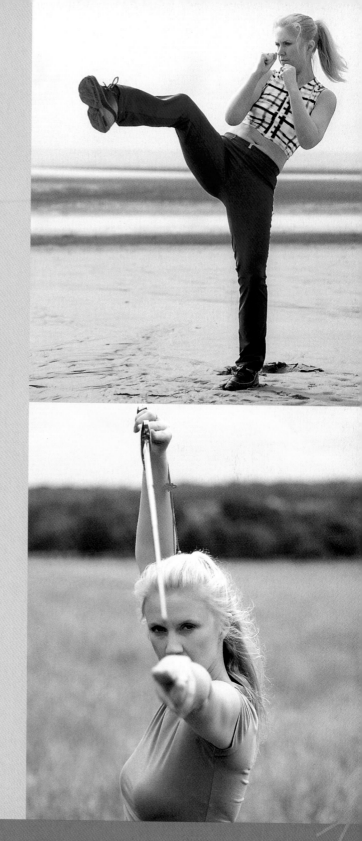

PENTJAK SILAT

In Indonesia, weapons and fighting arts are as old as the history of man. There are as yet too many gaps between historically proven facts and time to completely understand the meaning of the combative culture of this vast and diverse land. For an in-depth and accurate history of the martial arts of Indonesia read *The Weapons and Fighting Arts of Indonesia* by Donn F. Draegar (Charles E. Tuttle Company).

Aspects of all the above martial arts are covered in the workouts in this book. However there are many more discplines in which you can find classes quite easily

JU JITSU

The art of ju jitsu is interpreted as being the 'science of softness'. Translated literally, 'ju' means 'soft' or 'gentle' and

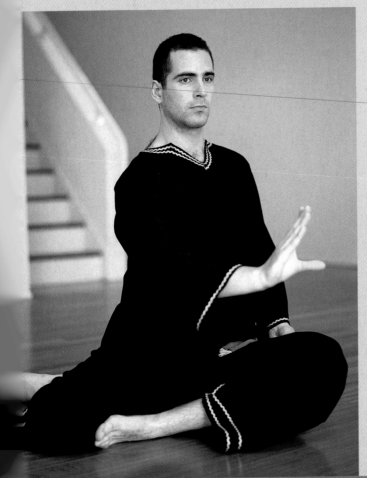

'jitsu' means 'art'. Whilst referred to as 'a gentle art' some of the techniques taught are extremely dynamic and would appear to be anything but soft.

There are many stories regarding the origins of ju jitsu, dating as far back as the eighth century, and some even claim it goes back to before the time of Christ. While some people claim that it originated in China, the ancient chronicles of Japan hold reference to early 'empty hand' techniques. It is believed, however, that ju jitsu was brought to Japan by a Chinese monk called Chen Yuanein (1587–1671). So, although ju jitsu is viewed today as a Japanese martial art, there is strong evidence pointing to Chinese origins.

While ju jitsu was first practised in Japan by the Samurai, followed by the Ninja, it inevitably spread further afield and was, unfortunately, embraced by many of the bandits of the time. Through this dubious and unwanted association, ju jitsu earned a poor reputation. It was during this period that Jiguro Kano developed the art of judo, (meaning 'the gentle way'), from a combination of ju jitsu techniques. His aim was to correct the reputation that ju jitsu had acquired as a deadly art through its unsavoury connections.

The central philosophy behind ju jitsu is to conquer an opponent by all and any means – as long as minimal force is used. A variation which is gaining popularity is Brazilian ju jitsu. This emphasises ground fighting – practitioners believe that since most fights end up on the ground, you might as well learn the most effective ground fighting techniques available.

The introduction of ju jitsu to Brazil is largely credited to Mitsuyo Maeda, who emigrated to Brazil in the 1920s and taught ju jitsu to Carlos Gracie of Rio de Janeiro. The large number of Japanese immigrants to South America (after all, the president of Peru is of Japanese ancestry) ensured that traditional martial arts, including ju jitsu, would find a home in Latin America. Brazilian ju jitsu evolved into its own distinct style honed in the rough favelas of the big cities, and no description of it is complete without mentioning the rest of the Gracie family. Carlos Gracie, after learning ju jitsu from Maeda, taught the art to his brothers Osvaldo, Gastao, Jorge and Helio. The Gracie family, through challenge matches, televised tournaments, and sheer numbers, have spread their namesake style throughout the world.

BRUCE LEE AND JEET KUNE DO   >>

No book on martial arts is complete without a mention of Bruce Lee, and the martial arts teaching that is his legacy. Lee was born in San Francisco in 1940, the son of a famous Chinese opera singer. They moved to Hong Kong where he became a child star in the growing film industry. His first film was *The Birth of Mankind*, and his last, uncompleted at the time of his death, *Game of Death*.

Lee was a loner and constantly getting into fights, and he looked towards kung fu as a way of disciplining himself. The famous Yip Men taught Lee his basic skills, but it was not long before he was mastering the master. At the age of nineteen Lee left Hong Kong to study philosophy at the University of Washington in the United States. He took a job as a waiter and also began to teach some of his skills to paying students.

Initially, Lee used the term jun fan gung fu, a development of the Wing Chun gung fu that he learned in Hong Kong, but came up against problems when dealing with larger Americans. This forced him to re-evaluate his art and he started to integrate boxing and fencing techniques and concepts into the Wing Chun. He also developed a grappling method put together from his training with leading experts of the day.

His unique methods led to many leading martial arts experts training with him and, in essence, learning how to fight all over again. Lee tore up the rule book, much to many people's displeasure. His jun fan style had certain unique features; it put the strongest hand to the fore and integrated trapping into kickboxing. His theories on timing and distance, developed from fencing, made his art unique.

His development of jeet kune do (JKD) came later. He believed that the technique approach of jun fan gung fu was flawed. JKD was a conceptual approach in which Lee sought to view the art of combat through principles, not techniques. From these principles he could develop a thousand techniques.

In 1970, Lee sustained a severe injury to his back. His doctors ordered him discontinue any martial training, and to remain in bed to allow his back to heal. In was at this time, whilst lying flat on his back for six months, that he began to write down his philosophies. The book, *The Tao of Jeet Kune Do*, remained unfinished at the time of his death. However it is one of the great martial arts works, and anyone who has ever been interested in not just Bruce Lee, but martial arts in general should be sure to read it.

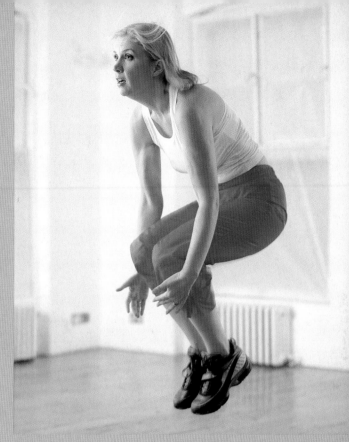

TAE KWON DO

Tae kwon do (TKD) is derived from several martial arts, its main influence being tae-kyon – Korean kick fighting. 'Tae' means 'to kick' or 'smash with the feet'; 'kwon' means 'to intercept' or 'to strike with the hands', and 'do' means 'the way of the art'. So the foundation of this martial art is to use both hands and feet to swiftly overcome your attacker.

TKD's origins stretch back over 2000 years and it is now practised by over 18 million people world-wide. It is an art of great range and contrast and includes breathtaking leaping and flying kicks, originally evolved to enable a fighter on foot to unseat a warrior on horseback.

At TKD clubs trainees follow basic training on stance and guard, learning various movements including blocks, punches, strikes and kicks. As training progresses the patterns of stance become more diversified and complicated, allowing simultaneous execution of two movements or more from the same position. This develops speed, power and flexibility.

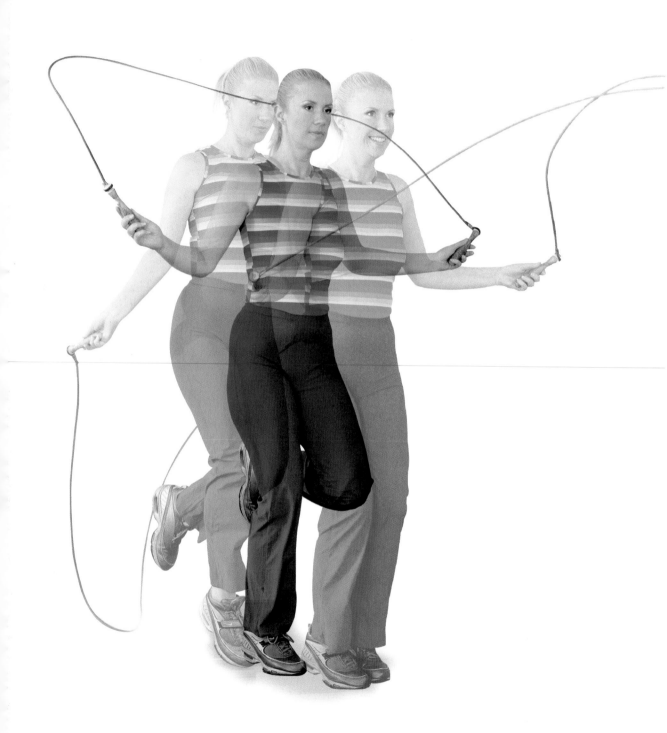

You are what you eat. You have probably heard this a thousand times, but how many times have you sat down and thought about it in the context of your fitness programme?

For us to get the most out of our workouts we need to be running on premium fuel, and that means a good, well-balanced diet. And note that 'diet' here does not mean a 'low-fat, eat-as-much-grapefruit-as-you-like-but-nothing-else, starvation plan', simply 'everything you eat and drink in the course of your daily life'.

FOOD AND EXERCISE >>

It is not easy to stick to any rigid dietary plan, no more so than it is to stick to one form of exercise, so it is important to have a basic understanding of what constitutes good nutrition. Traditional Chinese Medicine teaches us to go with the flow when it comes to our daily food intake. It advocates eating fresh food, in season, and keeping additives to a minimum. The seasons have an effect on everybody's life, wherever they live and whatever their age, lifestyle or occupation. Whether we are aware of them or not, the seasons act as a constantly changing backdrop to our lives.

Towards healthy eating

For most people, eating more healthily means making a few changes. Changing your eating habits is almost always a slow process. The worst mistake is to assume you can do it overnight – this rarely works and just leads to disillusionment. A slow change tends to be far more permanent than throwing over everything you are used to in favour of a brand new regime. By slowly weaning yourself off a packet of biscuits a day and replacing it with fruit, you might even come to prefer the latter (though we all need the occasional treat!). Start slowly and start to broaden the range of foodstuffs you buy. Experiment with different recipes and combinations of food. Your goal here is to find foods not only that you enjoy but that also make you feel good inside and out.

Here are a few pointers and ideas for healthy and seasonal eating – but remember, these are merely suggestions. Use these as a general guideline. Some might work for you, and others not. It is up to you to find out what works best for you and what makes you feel at the peak of health.

CARBS RULE !

One of the most common misconceptions is that all carbohydrates are fattening. Actually they are the best thing to eat for both physical and emotional balance, provided, of course, they are complex carbohydrates – unrefined grains, vegetables and fruits (bet you didn't think they could be carbs) and pulses all eaten in as natural a state as possible. Starches such as wheat or brown rice which have not been milled to death and still contain most of their natural minerals, fibre and vitamins, when consumed with fresh vegetables, provide a steady stream of energy.

Vegetables are fantastic things. Why? Because they have loads of powerful health-enhancing properties, which is why diets high in fresh vegetables are recommended against degenerative diseases such as cancer and arthritis. It is also important to make sure a lot of your vegetables are eaten raw. Traditional Chinese Medicine suggests you go about this process slowly. This is because raw foods are very effective cleansers, and if the body contains many toxins the cleansing reaction can be very powerful. It is best to start gently, so eat plenty of home-made vegetable soups, lightly steamed vegetables and stir-fries. Fresh vegetables are also a rich source of natural fibre, vitamins and minerals and they heighten your resistance to illness. Plenty of reasons to start scoffing more vegetables.

FIGHTING THE FAT

Some basic information about fat – did you know it prevents your body from making efficient use of carbohydrates and can encourage the development of diabetes? It also raises fat and cholesterol levels in your blood as well as uric acid, which contributes to the onset of gout, arthritis and arteriosclerosis. Finally a high-fat diet is believed to be a substantial factor in premature ageing and degenerative diseases. Do I need to go on?

There are two kinds of fat out there: saturated and unsaturated. Saturated fats in milk products and meat are basically useless except as a way of laying down more fat on your hips and belly (and not too many of us want this). The rest – unsaturated fats – are found in the processed oils you find on supermarket shelves such as sunflower and olive oil. They are also in margarines and convenience foods. Most have been chemically altered so your body cannot make use of the essential fatty acids they once contained. This can lead to fatty-acid deficiencies – so avoid them.

Having said all that, fat is an essential part of a healthy diet. Certain types of unsaturated fats are essential to the human body because they play an important part in maintaining the health of our immune system. Try to get your fat intake in the form of fatty fish (salmon for example) and cold-pressed, good-quality oils. We should be consuming 30–35 per cent of our daily calorie intake from 'good' fats.

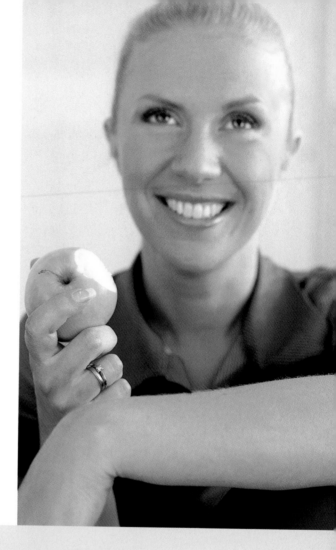

PROTEIN POINTERS

The belief that we need to eat protein in the form of meat as to stay healthy is misplaced. Studies show that a mixed diet of grains, roots, vegetables and fruits is a very good source of high-quality protein rather than our traditional meat, fish and dairy products which are high in fat and too concentrated in protein. So although we need to eat protein on a daily basis to help keep our cells topped up with amino acids , we need to pay particular attention to the source of that protein. Eat meat, fish and game by all means if you want to but do so in small quantities. Remember that some vegetables that you eat contain a good source of protein (peas for example) as do cereal grains such as barley, oats

above Healthy eating plays a vital role in any fitness regime. You can start by replacing your daily chocolate biscuits with fruit.

and rice. Our daily protein intake should be 10–12 per cent of our overall calorie intake. A bowl of chillied kidney beans eaten with a piece of corn bread or a peanut butter sandwich gives a good dose of your daily protein needs.

TAP WATER OR MINERAL WATER?

Natural spring water, tested for its quality and uncontaminated by chemical additives is one thing; the stuff flowing from your taps is another. Far from promoting your good health, it may be damaging it, due to the chemical pollutants it may contain. If you don't wish to buy bottled water then invest in a water filter; at least you know you are getting the pure thing.

WONDERFUL WATER

These days most of us know that we should be glugging water throughout the day, but we rarely get round to it. In fact we should be taking a slurp of water every fifteen minutes or so. Water is arguably one of the most important nutrients, not least of all because around 60 per cent of our body is water. Besides helping to regulate body temperature, it is the solvent for nutrients and wastes stored in your tissues which it can help to eliminate quickly and easily. Being dehydrated can slow down our metabolism and therefore energy generation making our muscles feel tired. We lose around 2.5 litres of water a day AT REST, and if you have being doing any form of exercise, say for example an hour's walk, you can lose another 1–2 litres.

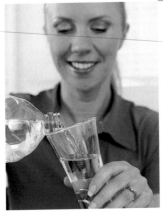

Some water replacement comes from our food. Fruit and vegetables, for example, have a very high water content in addition to their other attributes. We can probably get around 1–1.5 litres a day this way, which still leaves a considerable amount that needs to be replaced daily. One point to remember is that even if you have a large fluid intake each day, certain drinks such as tea, coffee, alcohol and many soft drinks (particularly those containing caffeine) are diuretics, and can actually accelerate water loss from the body

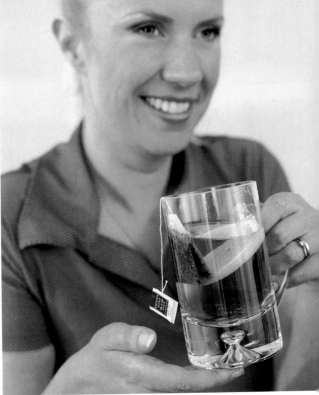

CANCEL THAT COFFEE!

One of the best things you can give up to help improve your health is coffee. Coffee contains caffeine and caffeine, unfortunately, is a drug. One of the xanthine group of chemicals, it stimulates the central nervous system, pancreas and heart as well as the cerebral cortex, making you feel temporarily more alert. However studies have shown that, while coffee drinking makes you feel more alert and efficient, in reality it impedes your mental performance. As with everything you cannot be expected to change your coffee drinking habits straight away. Start by cutting down every other cup and replacing it with herbal and fruit teas or mineral water. Soon drinking less and less coffee will become second nature and you should start feeling the benefits reasonably quickly. However you must remember that if you are a steady user of coffee, it is addictive, and you could have withdrawal symptoms. These can appear in the form of headaches or nausea, but are short-lived and well worth going through to rid your body of the caffeine once and for all.

AVOID ALCOHOL?

Alcohol, like caffeine and nicotine, is a drug. If taken over a long period of time, it can seriously damage your mind and body. It adversely affects the specific centres of the brain that govern judgement, self-control and personal inhibitions and to cap it all, the detrimental effects of alcohol on health and good looks are felt by the social drinker as well as the alcoholic.

Liver-cell damage and the increase in fat in the liver may be reversible if the drinker abstains from alcohol for long enough. But long-term damage to the liver resulting from daily consumption of alcohol over years can be irreversible.

The good news is that recent research has shown that a glass or two of red wine each day may lower the risk of a heart attack. The tannins in red wine help to prevent blood platelet cells from clumping together and triggering a heart attack. However much of the credit goes to the red pigments in the grape skins – so try red grapes or blueberries instead. The best advice is to drink sensibly and have nights off.

SLOW DOWN ON SALT

The recommended daily amount of sodium is about 3 grams a day. Many of us consume three or four times that amount. The small quantity that we require is available naturally in foods – vegetables, meats and fish, fruits and grains – without ever having to add salt to our foods.

Excess salt intake can severely upset the body's water balance and aggravate high blood pressure in those who have an inherited tendency towards it. We not only need to cut down on salt added during cooking but also to avoid many processed foods, such as canned vegetables, cooked meats, sauces and pickles, as these also contain high levels of salt.

ALL ABOUT SUGAR

Sugar is everywhere (some people's idea of heaven). It's in our chocolate bars, cereals, alcohol, milk and fruit in one form or other. It is common knowledge that the consumption of refined sugar has been linked with the development of degenerative illnesses. Eating sugar tends to raise your blood sugar levels and put stress on your pancreas, challenging it to maintain normal blood sugar levels. Sugar can also make you tired, depressed and emotionally unstable due to the insulin resistance and raised blood sugar levels triggered in your body. Here's your guide to where most common sugars come from.

>> Raw sugar, which is light tan in colour, is a coarse, granulated solid sugar that results when sugar cane is evaporated.

>> Refined sugar. Also known as table sugar or sucrose, this common sugar is found in the stalks of sugar cane and in the roots of sugar beet as a sugar-rich juice, which is extracted and then processed into dried sugar crystals.

>> Fruit sugar. Also known as fructose, fruit sugars are found naturally in all fruits, but they are also added to foods in the form of high-fructose corn syrup. Fructose is 1½ times sweeter than table sugar.

>> Brown sugar. This sugar is merely sugar crystals flavoured with molasses.

Out of all the sugars above, the best way to eat it is in a piece of fresh fruit.

Healthy Eating Guidelines

So to re-cap:

- Decrease daily fat intake to 30 per cent of your total daily calorie intake.

- Decrease intake of saturated (animal) fat to 25 per cent of your total daily calorie intake.

- Eat less animal protein.

- Eat more complex carbohydrates.

- Eat less sugar.

- Eat more fruit and vegetables.

- Decrease salt intake.

- Drink more water and cut down on caffeine-based drinks and alcohol.

- Add VARIETY to your daily diet.

Seasonal eating ideas

Cold winter days keep us inside craving comforting and hearty food. Spring emerges begging us to throw off the cobwebs and as bulbs start to pop up so does a huge variety of fresh green leaves. By the warm days of summer, nature has provided us with summer fruits to help keep us quenched and re-freshed. Eating seasonally also means eating what is available locally. Even in big

SPRING FOODS

Coming out of the darker days of winter into lighter longer days gives us a rise in our energy levels. Since we have probably been indulging in long-cooked warming dishes throughout the colder months, it is now time to throw off our winter cocoons and start looking forward to brighter days and lighter foods. In years gone by, there were very few fresh green vegetables available in the winter and people finished the winter months deficient in Vitamin C and iron. Though this is not so true today, there is still an increase of edible fresh leaves during the spring months. Eggs and dairy products are traditionally the foods of spring because this was the time of the year that hens began laying and cows producing milk. Eggs and milk are both perfect for making light meals. Forget about winter cabbages and try tender shoots of kale, broccoli, spinach, dark spring greens and cauliflowers. Later in the season there are spring cabbages, and leeks that can be used as an alternative to onions.

The best salad vegetable around is watercress which, at this time of year, has large leaves that are an excellent source of Vitamin C and iron. Try lightly steaming your vegetables to preserve as many vitamins as possible.

SUMMER FOODS

Summer gives a plenitude of choice, providing us with an enormous variety of fruits and vegetables in quick succession. However, since their shelf life is short, we need to enjoy them quickly. During the longer, warmer days we need cooling foods such as soft summer fruits and leafy salads. Combine these with high-energy grain foods such as pasta, rice and couscous – think fresh tomato sauces and pasta with a green salad.

Lettuces and radishes are the first to arrive and can be picked throughout the summer months. Spring onions and cucumbers are not too far behind to help make fantastic salads. Then there's asparagus, broad beans and peas, followed closely by new potatoes, small sweet carrots and beetroot. Added to this list as the summer progresses are courgettes, marrows, tomatoes, French beans, peppers and aubergines – we really are spoilt for choice.

Summer fruits start with the smaller berries – gooseberries, redcurrants and blackcurrants. Strawberries and raspberries follow. Try one of my favourite dishes – raspberries mixed with redcurrants with a dash of orange juice and a sprinkle of fructose. Leave to marinate for a couple of hours and eat with yoghurt.

After that come various types of cherries from the smaller English yellow ones to large succulent Morellos. In the late summer there are plums and blackberries and the first apples of the season (think apple and blackberry pies and baked apples with cinnamon).

cities, farmer's markets are now a regular sight, so freshly grown fruit and vegetables are more easily available. You could even consider growing your own. Even one or two tomato plants in the back garden are better than nothing. Organic meat is also now widely available. You can even order off the Internet and get fresh organic meats delivered straight to your front door.

AUTUMN FOODS

Early autumn continues with summer's abundance. The days can remain warm, but the evenings start to draw in and get cooler. Now is the time to make hot fulfilling dishes using the last of the summer's vegetables. Think soups, potato-based meals and grilled vegetable dishes. Potatoes come into their own at this time of year and are the most versatile of foods. The first nuts start to come into the shops. These autumn nuts, such as walnuts and cobnuts, have a fresh-tasting and milky texture and flavour completely different to the winter ones.

At the beginning of autumn there are still tomatoes, peppers, aubergines, marrows, runner beans and courgettes. Soon there will be sweetcorn, pumpkins and different varieties of winter squashes. Jerusalem artichokes, swede, turnips and celeriac are also ready. And onions are now at their best, so try button and pickling onions which are great in stews and casseroles. Apples and pears in many varieties are the autumn's main fruits. There will also be the last of plums, raspberries and blackberries. Try pears poached in red wine with cloves, nutmeg and almonds.

WINTER FOODS

Cold frosty days make us want to hibernate and put on some winter warmth (unfortunately, sometimes in more ways than one), and cooking becomes an excellent pastime. Warming, energy-giving foods are needed during these months and root vegetables, with their bulk and richness, are ideal. This is the time of year to get baking. Not only is bread a fantastic high-energy food but there are also so many varieties to be made. The added bonus is the all-pervasive smell of freshly baked bread – who can resist? Seasonal winter vegetables are the root vegetables, such as carrot, parsnip, swede and celeriac. Potatoes are still excellent. Then there's the typical green vegetables of winter such as Brussels sprouts and Savoy cabbages. Apples and pears last well into the winter months and this is a perfect time of year to make use of dried fruits. Try a winter salad of grated carrots, grated apples, radishes, apple juice and crushed garlic with a drizzle of extra-virgin olive oil.

HOW TO EAT!

Small amounts and often. Instead of three large meals a day, try splitting it into four or five smaller ones. This gives the body constant fuelling throughout the day and avoids the strain of suddenly digesting large amounts of food.

ROOT OUT THE RUBBISH

Open your kitchen cupboards and take a good hard look. Then get a box or a binbag and chuck everything into it that doesn't agree with your new-found principles. Jams and spreads? Replace with a variety that doesn't contain any sugar or preservatives. They are delicious and much better for you. Jars of coffee? Replace with herbal or fruit teas. White rice and pasta? Replace with whole-wheat. If you really can't bear chucking it or giving it away, then use it up. Just remember to re-adjust your shopping habits.

below A few minutes of rest and relaxation before sitting down to eat will greatly improve both your enjoyment and your digestive processes.

EAT BEFORE OR AFTER EXERCISE?

Eating within the hour before strenuous exercise is never a good idea. However if you are going to exercise first thing in the morning, don't do so on an empty stomach. In the same way that you wouldn't try and drive your car if it had no petrol in it, you shouldn't make your body work when it has been fasting all night. A banana-based smoothie or yoghurt drink packed with fruit is an excellent source of energy and not too heavy on the stomach. The optimum time to replace lost energy is within 2 hours of exercising – the body just loves and gobbles up carbohydrates. Have a portion of carbohydrates weighing roughly 50 grams. This could be a large baked potato, 2 large bananas, 225 grams of cooked pasta or a 250-gram pack of mixed dried fruit.

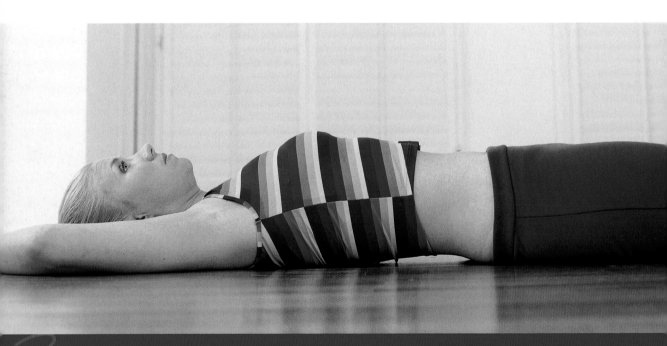

HAPPY THOUGHTS

Try and eat meals in the right frame of mind; in other words, do not sit down to a meal if you feel cross or frustrated. Calm down and relax before you eat. Enjoy the whole experience of eating – the smell, the look and the taste are all equally important. Also beware of comfort eating; the next time someone or something has annoyed you, try not to take it out on three bars of chocolate. You never really enjoy food in this frame of mind and usually just end up feeling more cross with yourself.

right Try to cultivate a relaxed frame of mind before eating, but avoid vigorous exercise too close to a meal. Yoga is ideal.

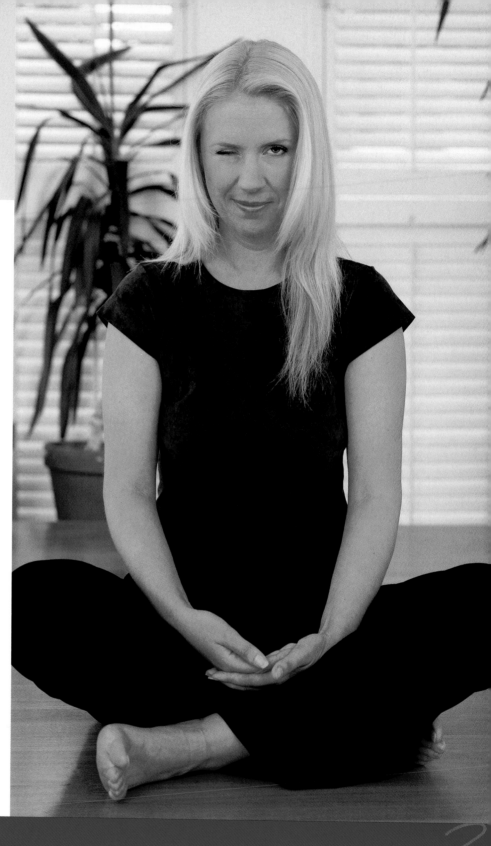

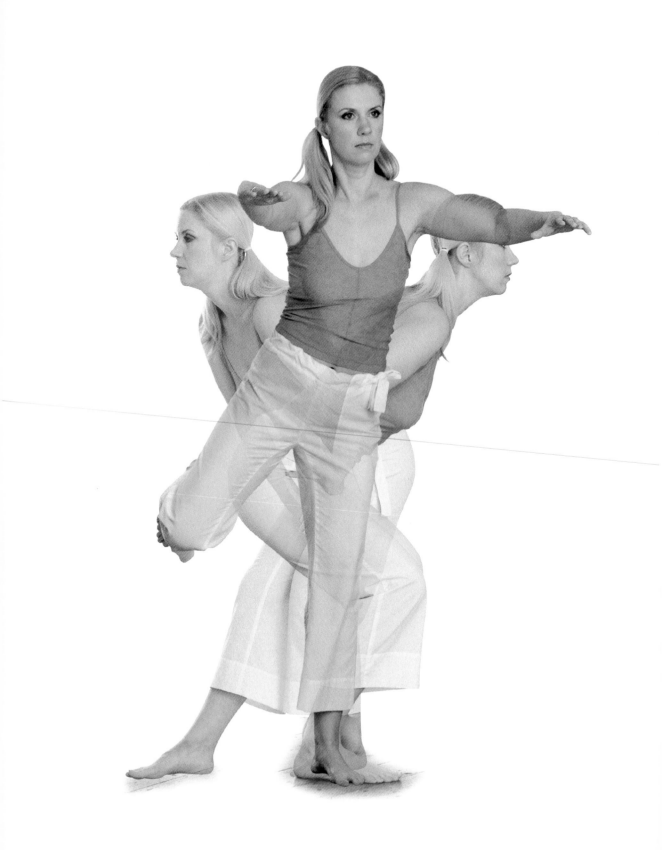

*'If I had six hours to chop down a tree,
I'd spend the first four hours sharpening the axe.'*
ABRAHAM LINCOLN

Visualise a tree. Immediately we think of a solid trunk with leafy branches sprouting forth. This tree will withstand hail, sleet, snow and wind because deep in the ground it has put down a solid base of roots. The foundation stone of all our workouts lies in the essential warming up and cooling down components. Without these we are failing to prepare

BUILDING A FOUNDATION >>

ourselves, both physically and mentally, for the main body of work. During the warm-up phase, the body adapts to the increased blood and oxygen flow to the heart and other muscles. Mentally we are becoming focused on the workout ahead, letting everyday distractions slip aside and beginning to concentrate on the forthcoming exercises.

Similarly, the heart, even though a strong and efficient muscle, needs a gentle cool-down period to allow its rate drop slowly and safely. As the heart rate gently increases during the warm-up, the cool-down involves a series of decreasingly easy moves. Think of slowing down from a sprint to a fast run, through a jog and into a walk. All cool-downs and workouts should finish with a thorough stretch.

So how do I warm-up?

There are various different methods of warming up but the main rule is to start off slowly and build up gradually. The basic warm-up should last at least five minutes before the body is physically warm enough to go through the initial stretches. There are several aerobic options. If you have the inclination (and weather permits) walking is an excellent way. A walk around the block, starting off at an average daily pace and then building up to a very brisk walk, is a simple and effective option.

Many of us have redundant exercise equipment, such as exercise bikes, steppers or rowers, lying around the house gathering dust. Drag it out, wipe it down and use it! If it hasn't been used in a considerable period of time, it is advisable to check that it is in safe working order. The same principle applies as for the options above when using exercise equipment – start slowly and build up gradually. If neither of the above options appeals, put on some music and follow these basic aerobic moves.

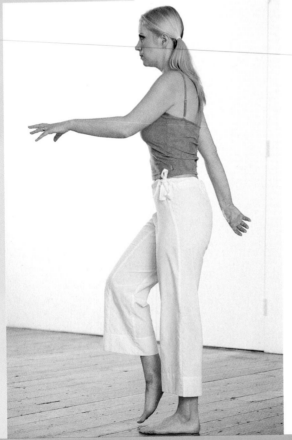

WARM-UP WORKOUT

<< **Marching** – Start off on the spot and then move forwards and backwards. Keep the feet softly flexed and don't slam them down. Keep your back straight and your abdominal muscles tight. Use your arms, keeping the elbows bent and the fists soft, and pump your arms as you march. *Continue for at least one minute.*

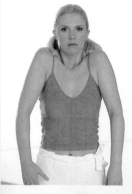

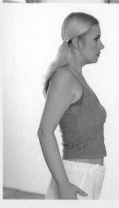

Heel digs – Moving on from the march, place alternate heels to the front, keeping the foot flexed. Punch your arms out straight in front. Keep the supporting knee soft and the back straight. *Continue for at least one minute.*

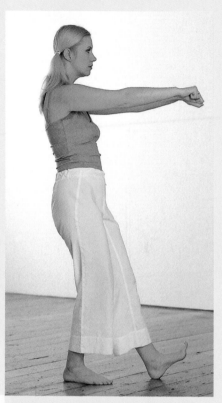

Shoulder rolls – Keep marching throughout this move. Using their fullest range of motion, gently roll your shoulders forwards five times and backwards five times. Let your arms hang loose by your sides and just let your shoulders do the work.

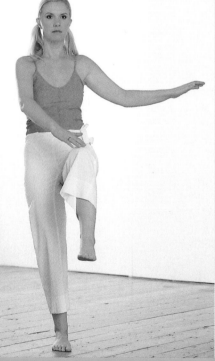

Knee lifts – Now bring up each knee to touch the alternate hand. Don't lean forwards or backwards. Keep the abdominal muscles tight and the back straight. Again make sure your supporting knee is not locked. *Continue for at least one minute.*

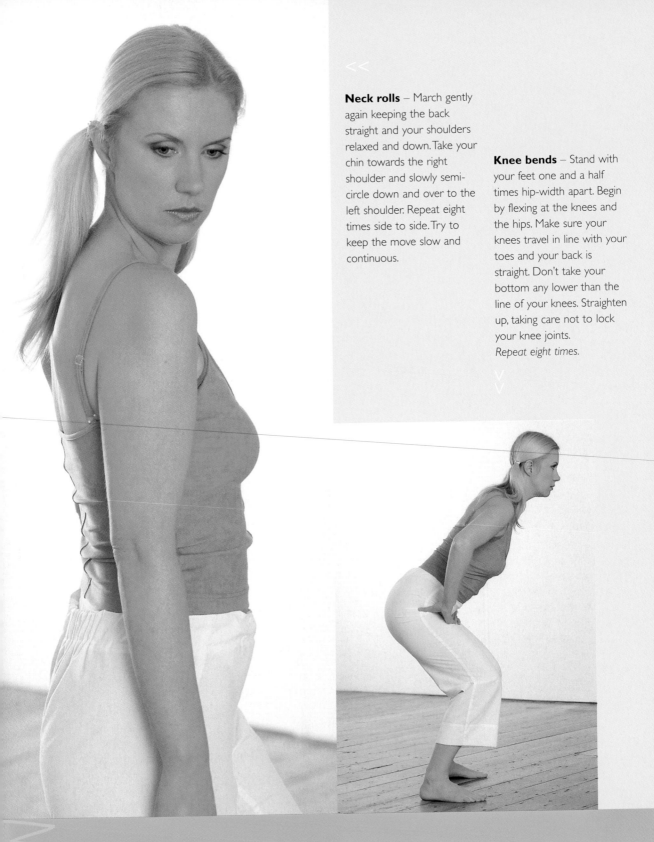

Neck rolls – March gently again keeping the back straight and your shoulders relaxed and down. Take your chin towards the right shoulder and slowly semi-circle down and over to the left shoulder. Repeat eight times side to side. Try to keep the move slow and continuous.

Knee bends – Stand with your feet one and a half times hip-width apart. Begin by flexing at the knees and the hips. Make sure your knees travel in line with your toes and your back is straight. Don't take your bottom any lower than the line of your knees. Straighten up, taking care not to lock your knee joints. *Repeat eight times.*

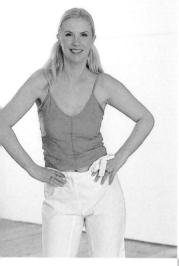

Side steps – Step side to side now with long easy strides. Place the feet down toes first, heels following. Keep the body upright and the head lifted. Start with your hands on your hips and then begin to push the hands out in front every other stride.
Continue for at least one minute.

Leg curls – Add to the side steps by bringing alternate heels up towards your bottom. Make sure your supporting knee is always soft and don't slam your feet down.
Continue for at least one minute.

Pelvic circles– Stand with your feet hip-width apart, with the knees soft and back straight. Place your hands on your hips and gently circle your pelvis in a D-shape, straight across the back and around the front. Try to isolate the move purely to your hips, keeping the knees and upper body as still as possible.
Repeat five times in one direction then change and repeat the other way.

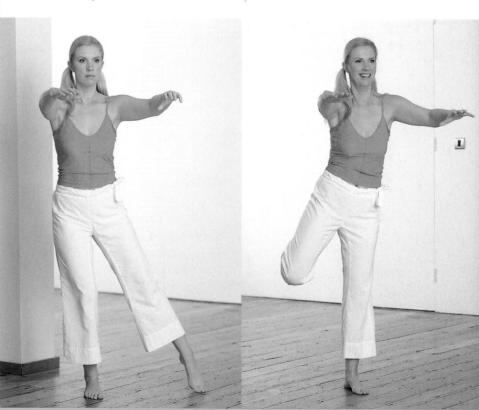

Warm-up stretches

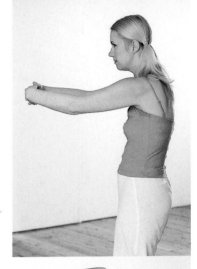

REMEMBER TO:

>> HOLD EACH
STRETCH FOR ABOUT
10 SECONDS

>> STRETCH TO A POINT
OF TENSION NOT PAIN

>> KEEP BREATHING
THROUGHOUT

Now the muscles are warm follow these short stretches for all-over body flexibility.

Top of back stretch (trapezius) – >>
Stand with feet hip-width apart and the knees slightly bent. Link the hands, with palms facing you, and reach out until you feel a stretch across the top of your back. Keep the elbows soft and the chin slightly down. Imagine you are hugging a beachball.

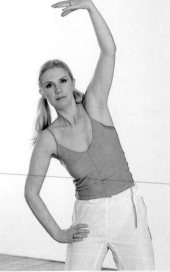

Back and waist stretch (latissimus dorsi and obliques) – >> Stand with your feet one and a half times hip-width apart and knees slightly bent. Lean to the right and reach up with the right hand. Then lean over to the left, supporting the torso with the opposite hand. Aim to feel the stretch all along the right side. Change sides.

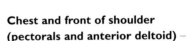

Chest and front of shoulder (pectorals and anterior deltoid) – >>
Clasp the hands together behind the back and then lift them slightly away from the body. Keep the elbows bent, back straight and abdominals tight. Aim to feel the stretch across the front of the chest.

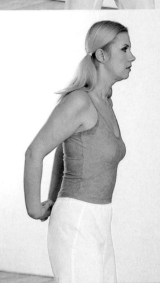

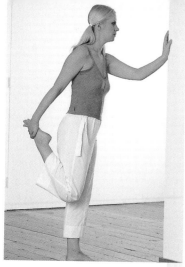

<< **Front of thigh (quadriceps)** – Use the wall for support if necessary. Keeping the back straight, flex the knee and grasp the ankle. Gently draw the heel to the bottom. Keep the supporting knee bent and try to keep the knees parallel. You should feel the stretch down the front of the bent thigh. Change legs.

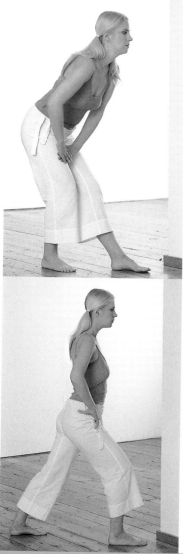

<< **Back of thigh (hamstring)** – Bend the left leg and extend the right one. Lean forwards keeping the right leg straight but the knee not locked. Place hands on left thigh. Aim to feel the stretch in the back of the right thigh. Keep your back straight and your abdominal muscles tight. Change legs.

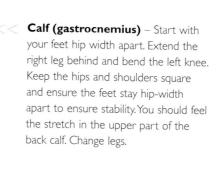

<< **Calf (gastrocnemius)** – Start with your feet hip width apart. Extend the right leg behind and bend the left knee. Keep the hips and shoulders square and ensure the feet stay hip-width apart to ensure stability. You should feel the stretch in the upper part of the back calf. Change legs.

THE COOL-DOWN WORKOUT

After exercise, always spend at least five minutes taking the heart rate slowly and safely down using exercises of decreasing intensity.

Spend 30–60 seconds doing each of the following:

- *Skipping on the spot*
- *Knee lifts with arms*
- *Knee lifts without arms*
- *Heel digs with bicep curls*
- *Heel digs with no arms*
- *Gentle marching on spot*

You can also use any of the warm-up options such as the home exercise equipment or walking, as part of a cool-down routine. Start at a moderate level and decrease the intensity until you feel you have returned to your normal daily state. Never skimp on cool-down. Even if you just walk around the house it is very important that you help your heart, lungs and muscles gradually slow down. Your muscles are now in prime condition to be stretched and flexed. The stretching component should always be followed through. If you need to shorten your workout, cut some out of the middle, never the beginning or the end. Use a stretching workout from chapter nine to help increase your body's flexibility and prevent any injuries.

What should I wear?

Your shoes are the most important item to consider whilst exercising. You should wear clothes you feel comfortable in and can move freely in. Ideally, wear layers of breathable fabrics which can be peeled off as your body temperature rises.

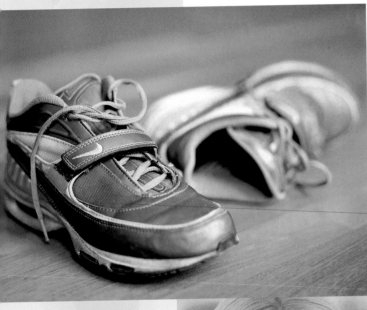

above Taking the time to choose the correct training shoes will pay dividends later.

Shoes needn't be the most expensive on the market, though do expect to pay in the region of £60.00 for a decent pair. Most training shoes need to be replaced after they have logged 400–500 miles of work, so if you are still wearing your old school gym shoes, now is the time to replace them. Even if you are not sure about the amount of wear left in your existing trainers, go and try on some new pairs. You will be surprised, in comparison, at the amount of support that a new pair gives. Spend time trying on various different makes of shoes and don't be afraid to jump up and down or run around in them (some larger shops have treadmills specifically for you to do this). Choose a cross trainer or a shoe designed for aerobic classes or gym work rather than a running shoe. These will be designed with good cushioning in the forefront and the heel, to lessen the impact during jumping, as well as offering lateral stability to help avoid injury to the ankles.

Shop for shoes at the end of the day or after a workout when your feet are generally at their largest. Wear the type of socks you usually wear during exercise, and if you use orthotic devices (inserts) for your feet, make sure you wear them when trying on shoes. Finally remember regardless of style, fit is the most important consideration. Don't be swayed by fashion. No matter how good you hear a shoe is, no matter how good it looks, if it doesn't fit you or you are not comfortable with it, don't buy it.

Where shall I exercise?

The majority of people who buy fitness books intend to use them within the privacy of their own home, but this is not set in stone. Most of the workouts contained within this book can be happily translated to the garden, the local park or beach. In fact, in my mind, there is nothing nicer than exercising outdoors.

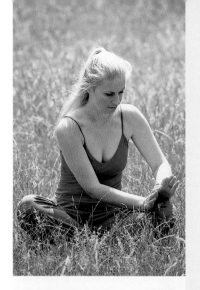

I have discovered that people fall into two very definite camps, those that will go outside at a drop of a hat, and those that are pulled kicking and screaming into the great outdoors. It is quite simply a personal preference. However if you've never tried a jog along a sunny beach or done tai chi whilst watching a magnificent sunrise, then at least give it a go. At home, most of us have one room (with a small amount of rearrangement) that has enough space to work out in. A full length mirror is useful for checking technique and you might want to add something to play music on. Finally a decent skipping rope and a set of small handweights weighing 1–2lb (500g–1kg), available from most sport shops or department stores, will be useful but not entirely necessary.

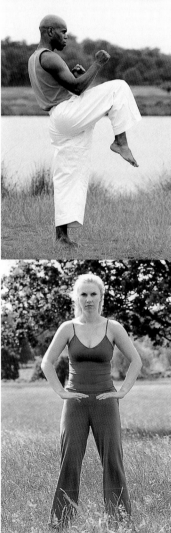

right Exercising in the open air can enormously increase your feeling of well-being, especially if, like many people, you spend much of your day cooped up indoors.

Do I need a fitness evaluation before I start an exercise programme?

Perhaps. If you haven't been exercising regularly and have any of the following characteristics, you should consult your doctor before starting this or any other exercise routine.

- Have you ever been diagnosed with a **heart condition**, or is there a history of heart disease in the family?
- Are you more than three stone (42lb) **overweight**?
- Do you have **high blood pressure**?
- Are you **diabetic**?
- Are you **asthmatic** or do you have a history of breathing problems?
- Are you **pregnant** or trying to become pregnant?
- Have you recently **given birth**?
- Have you had **surgery** in the last six weeks?
- Have you recently experienced **chest pain** during physical activity?
- Have you a **high cholesterol** level?

- Have you ever been advised by a doctor to **avoid exercise**?
- Do you need to see a **physiotherapist**?

As we see in chapter nine, The Healing Hand, most of us tend to view physiotherapists and related professionals as people we turn to when we have become injured or are in pain. However, it is important to view them as a preventative measure too. Have a look at the following questions, if you answer 'yes' to any of them, it is worth booking a consultation before you start this or any other exercise programme.

- Have you ever fractured or broken any **bones**?
- Do you have **bunions** or other foot problems?
- Do you suffer from **knee pain**?
- Have you ever had **shin splints**?
- Do you suffer from **lower back problems**?
- Do you suffer **regular twinges** in your shoulders or upper back muscles?
- Have you had any surgery on a **joint or ligaments**?
- Have you ever been told **not to exercise** for any length of time by a relevant professional such as a physiotherapist?

Some helpful hints!

Don't be put off by the fear of looking stupid. Failure is an integral part of everyone's learning process. If you don't feel you are getting it right, try to become aware of your mistakes and then do it again. Remember, practice makes perfect.

Working out with a friend is a great motivator. Not only can you watch and learn from each other's new-found techniques, but you also have a training partner who can encourage you on less enthused days.

Learn to enjoy getting the techniques as correct as possible. One of the joys and benefits of martial arts is the increased results you get out of practising the basics. Repeating the same technique might seem like a waste of time, but learning to

appreciate the nuance of every move will markedly improve the quality of your workout. By recognising that everything has natural stages to it – we learn to walk before we run – we become mentally prepared to thoroughly learn basic skills.

The basics

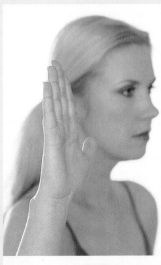

<< HOW TO MAKE A FIST

- Spread out all your fingers
- Begin folding in from the tops of the fingers leaving out the thumb. Fold the fingers over and clench them into the palm.
- Place thumb firmly upon the four folded fingers.
- Keep your fist strong and tight, but not so tense that you feel strain in your forearm or wrist. The striking point would be the front part of the index and middle finger.
- Don't grip too hard
- Don't wear rings or bracelets
- Watch out for long finger nails – they will dig into your palms

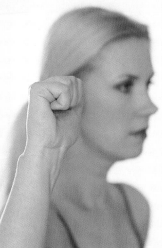

HOW TO PUNCH SAFELY

- Never extend your arm so far that you lock any joints.
- Keep your fist, wrist and elbow in perfect alignment so that they form an unbroken line throughout.
- Breathe out on every punch, and inhale as you retract.
- Visualise a target, then punch through it.
- Remember a punch is not just thrown from the arms and shoulders, it requires correct whole body mechanics to make it safe and effective.

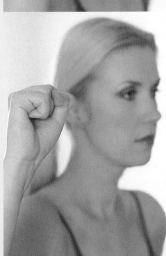

HOW TO KICK SAFELY

- Avoid overextended, far-reaching kicks that lock your joints.
- Keep the supporting knee soft.
- Breathe out as you kick, and inhale as you retract.
- Kick only to a height which feels comfortable for you.
- Learn the basic moves well; start with low kicks and work up.
- Keep your abdominal muscles tight as you kick.
- Don't slam the kicking foot down.
- Retract the kicking leg through its original path and place the foot down softly.
- Always visualise your imaginary target and look towards it.

How to use the workouts

However great it would be just to exercise when we felt like it, it is not necessarily going to give us much in the way of results. To achieve long-term health and fitness benefits we need to exercise three times a week. However this doesn't mean we need to stick to the same old routine week in and week out. In fact, the more we keep our fitness methods varied, the more likely we are to get fit and keep healthy. All of the workouts in this book can be done in conjunction with a normal fitness programme (such as going to the gym, bike riding or aerobic classes) or by themselves. I would especially like this book to inspire you to try various pure martial art classes. In giving you a taster and arming you with background knowledge of individual disciplines, I hope you will find it an exciting adventure to go and train in the martial arts world.

Setting goals

Before getting into some suggested workout routines, you need to start at the beginning. First, decide what you want to achieve, and then write it down. Setting goals and then keeping a training diary are the most important fitness tools next to pure willpower. Split your goals into the short and the long term. For example:

My short-term goals are:
• To exercise three times a week
• To eat more healthily
• To feel my tummy is less flabby

My long-term goals are:
• To be able to run for the bus without getting out of breath
• To lose my excess fat so I can happily wear a swimming costume.

To achieve the above goals you need to choose some workouts which are cardiovascular, to burn off calories and therefore fat, and some which are toning, for the abdominal muscles. You can buy special training diaries from sports shops but your own diary or kitchen calendar will do just as well. Sit down at the beginning of every week and plan when are the best times to exercise. Write it down and stick to it.

For maximum benefits decide what each workout is going to entail. Pick your workouts for the week, work out how much time they are going to take and write that down too. This sounds long winded but it it is worth it as it means you are less likely to give up halfway through a workout.

HERE IS AN EXAMPLE OF A TRAINING DIARY ENTRY:

Monday
- **Time** 30 minutes
- **Workout** Hi-chi Workout
- **Notes** Got up and took the dog for ½ hour brisk walk before work. Felt really invigorated so had a very healthy breakfast. Did Hi-chi workout in the garden after work – feel really pleased with myself for exercising twice in one day.

Tuesday
Rest day

Wednesday
- **Time** 1 hour
- **Workout** Balanced Body workout and stretch
- **Notes** Tried doing the workout before work, but don't feel I got much out of it (was worried about being late).
NB next time do it in the evening.

Thursday
Rest day

Friday
- **Time** 30 minutes
- **Workout** The Core Workout
- **Notes** Ended up going to the pub after work so no workout!

Saturday
- **Time** 1 hour
- **Workout** Stretches
- **Notes** Feeling hungover so went for an hour's brisk walk. Came home and stretched.

Sunday
Rest day

LET'S KEEP MOTIVATED!

It is very easy to come up with excuses not to exercise. You need to treat your workout routine as you would a relationship or your career, always look for new ways to keep it exciting, otherwise it will just fizzle out.

EASE INTO IT

If you haven't been following any exercise routine for a while, don't expect to bounce back immediately to your former fit self. Instead, ease yourself into exercise by starting off at a low intensity and gradually building up. Starting any form of exercise will inevitably cause some muscle soreness – you don't want to be in so much pain that your first attempt becomes your last.

JUST DO IT

Even professional athletes have to coax themselves into a workout once in a while. Getting started is always the toughest part. If you don't feel like exercising, tell yourself you will only do it for 10–15 minutes. Doing something is ALWAYS better than nothing. And the chances are that once you get started, you'll keep going.

KEEP IT NEW

Don't let yourself fall into the habit of doing the same exercise day in and month out. Not only will you get mentally bored but your fitness levels will 'plateau' and you will stop achieving anything. Try to make a year plan of other activities you would like to try – run a mini marathon, take up horse riding – and add that to your workouts.

INVOLVE YOUR FAMILY AND FRIENDS

Getting someone to exercise with you is always great. If no one seems that keen then at least ask them to keep you motivated. Pick someone supportive and then outline your goals. Having someone who knows what you should be doing is very helpful. At least you will be less likely to raid the biscuit tin in front of them.

Workout suggestions

Here are some of the most common goals, with suggested solutions for each. I have given suggestions for exercising on Mondays, Wednesdays and Fridays. Of course you don't have to stick to these days but you should try to exercise three times a week and make sure you have a day off in between exercising to let the muscles rest and recuperate.

cross references

p. 52   hi-chi workout
p. 109   abdominal workout
p. 115   silat workout
p. 118   lower-back workout
p. 153   stretches

'I would like to lose some of my excess body flab'	**Monday**	**Wednesday**	**Friday**
You need a cardiovascular (aerobic) workout to help burn off excess fat – combine this workout with a sensible healthy diet to combat excess calories and fight the fat on two fronts	Hi-chi workout	Brisk walk or walk/jog for 30 minutes	Hi-chi workout ★Bonus points for another brisk walk at the weekend (including quick stretch)
'Give me a flat tummy please' Flat tummies are achieved by toning the abdominal muscles. Work on your abdominal muscles and your lower back muscles to ensure balance. Most of us who desire that six pack already have it (honestly!) but it is hidden under a small layer of excess fat. Therefore to ensure great looking abs, you need a fat-burning workout too.	**Monday** Abdominal and lower back workout	**Wednesday** Hi-chi workout or brisk walk	**Friday** Silat workout or the same as Monday ★Bonus points for another brisk walk and/or jog at the weekend (include stretch)

'I never have enough
time to do anything....
I feel really stressed
AND really floppy'

First you need to get into the
right frame of mind – a short
stress-busting workout is the
priority. Follow this with an
'anti-floppy' workout which
includes all-over toning.

Monday
Mind Maze workout

Wednesday
Dao Yin exercise from
The De-stress Zone followed
by stretch from Healing Hand
chapter

Friday
All-over workout from Law of
Balance chapter

★Bonus points for either
  meditating or deep breathing
  any day of the week.

I want firmer thighs
and a smaller bum!'

One of the great quests of
life...firm thighs and small bottoms
is achieved by a combination of
toning, kicking and aerobic work.

Monday
Hi-chi workout

Wednesday
Lower-body workout
from Law of Balance
chapter

Friday
All-over workout from Law of
Balance chapter

★Bonus points for fitting in on the
  days in between
  a 30 minute fast walk

'I want to touch
my toes...'

This lack of flexibility is something
that, with simple application of the
right work, is easily remedied.
However it is not something that is
done quickly. Expect several
months of gentle stretching before
you see any huge results. Hang in
there though, it is worth it!

Monday
Quick all-over stretch from The
Healing Hand chapter

Wednesday
Hips and buttocks and legs and
knees stretches from The Healing
Hand chapter

Friday
Dao Yin workout from The De-
stress Zone followed by Quick all-
over stretch from Healing Hand
chapter.

★Bonus points for fitting in a quick
  stretch whenever you are warm.
  Just walked home from the
  shops? Fit that stretch in!

'My lower body is fine, but the backs of my arms are beginning to resemble bats' wings'

Another common problem. Flabby backs of arms can make us all feel hideous but a few months of working out using a combination of boxing and toning should help to tone them up in no time.

Monday
Upper-body workout from Law of Balance chapter

Wednesday
Hi-chi workout

Friday
Upper-body workout from Law of Balance chapter

'I can't sleep at night.... any suggestions?'

Working out late at night does not work for everybody, but working through a simple de-stress exercise may help.

Anytime
Try the Evening De-stress workout from The De-stress Zone followed by meditating or deep breathing any evening before bed.

cross references

p. 52 hi-chi workout
p. 62 upper-body workout
p. 70 lower-body workout
p. 78 all-over workout
p. 88 mind maze workout
p. 133 evening de-stress workout
p. 134 dao yin workout
p. 139 meditation
p. 153 stretches
p. 157 hips and buttocks stretch
p. 159 legs and knees stretch
p. 166 quick all-over stretch

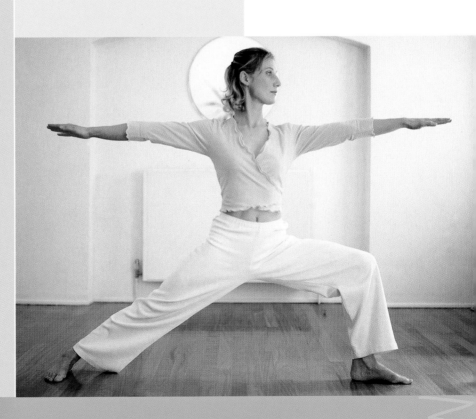

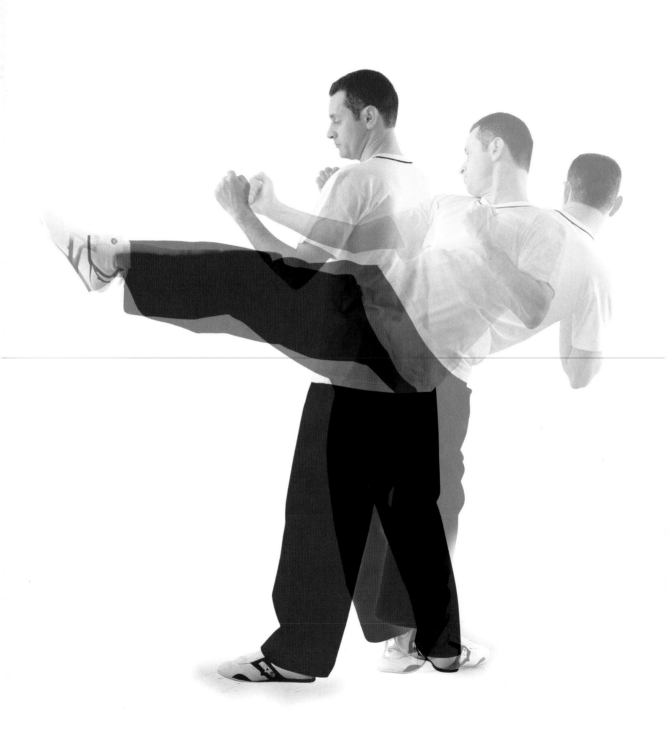

What is Chi? The Chinese call it 'Chi', the Japanese 'Ki' and in India it is known as 'Prana'. The closest Western translation becomes 'vital energy' or 'life force', which according to Eastern philosophies is present in all life. It is seen as the life energy within everything. It is not the breath itself; it is the breath which carries in the chi. Chi is present throughout the universe, and is shared and exchanged between all living beings and all matter in the universe. When this energy flows freely, the mind, body and spirit are alert and work harmoniously. When blocked, their function is inhibited and ill health can result.

WORKING WITH THE SPIRIT >>

Although it is fascinating to try to appreciate and understand chi intellectually and conceptually, it really must be felt – in the body, in the spirit and in the movement of the breath. Our Western way of thinking, of splitting the mind and body, can make it very difficult for us to comprehend chi. However in Eastern culture the union of mind and body is taken for granted. When studying Eastern disciplines, therefore, you have to work on intuition, on developing a better sensitivity to the truth of an experience and to the integrity of a person. It is all part of the discipline of martial arts. There are seven types of chi. By looking at each individually we can begin to understand how Eastern philosophies see how the health of the physical, mental and emotional are entwined.

BREATH CHI

The way in which air is inhaled and exhaled is as important as the quality and quantity of that air. Poor and incorrect breathing affects the functioning of the brain as well as the memory and concentration levels, emotional stability, heart, muscles, lungs, circulation and nervous system. Because oxygen is believed to be the engine of our chi, deep correct breathing is necessary when the flow of chi through the body needs re-stimulating.

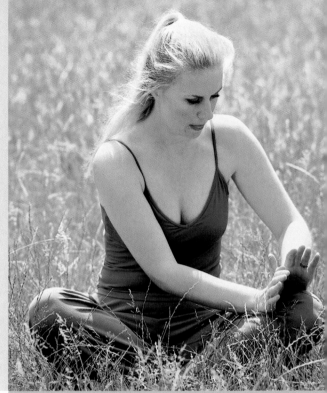

FOOD CHI

Food is another fundamental source of life force. The Chinese have an ancient tradition of taking great care to plan and prepare their meals in ways that preserve it. Vegetables are cut in a certain way (to imitate the direction of the flowing chi), and cooking is done over a flame (electricity and microwaving are believed to destroy chi). Traditional Chinese Medicine dictates that food should be eaten in season. For example, yang foods, such as vegetables that grow below the ground, fish and red meat are eaten in winter, whereas summer is the time to consume yin food such as light fish, white meat and vegetables grown above ground.

ORIGINAL CHI

The chi that we are born with is called original chi and comprises what we know as the 'constitution'. The quality of original chi can be partially predetermined by our parents' health at the time of our conception. Their general state of mental, physical and emotional health combined with other factors such as the quality of their diet and their age all combine to affect our original chi. Being born with weak chi can require constant effort throughout life, necessitating correct dietary habits, moderate exercise and proper breathing to sustain and invigorate the constitution. On the other hand, those lucky enough to be born with a strong constitution often take their good health for granted. It is easy to go through life abusing it until it is weakened and poor health results.

INTERNAL CHI

This is the chi upon which our internal body relies for its health and correct functioning. Internal chi flows with the blood to all our inner organs and through all our meridians, helping to keep our yin and yang energies shifting and our body balanced. Moderate amounts of sufficiently energetic daily movement and exercise are essential to keep our internal chi flowing freely.

EXTERNAL CHI

This type of energy is all around us, but can only be sensed and accessed by the very sensitive. For example, highly trained chi kung masters can read our bodies for signs of physical imbalance or disease. Alongside acupuncture and reiki, chi kung can be used to heal, recharge and rebalance an unwell organ.

NUTRITIVE CHI

This moves with the blood via the heart and blood vessels to deliver nourishment to our inner organs, cells, tissues, muscles and bones.

PROTECTIVE CHI

This protective chi helps the body to resist and expel infections that penetrate the natural lines of defence.

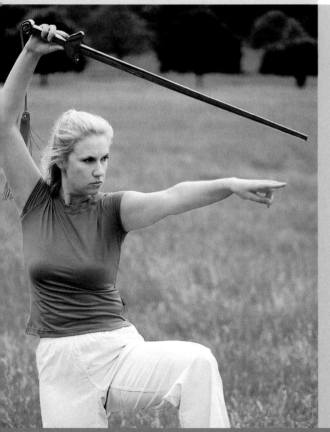

Finding a balance

All aspects of our health combine to create an overall feeling of total well-being. Whatever your beliefs, the principle of looking after all areas of your health makes perfect sense. There is no point physically exercising everyday, strengthening your body, if the stress of work causes a nervous breakdown. Everything should be considered in moderation and looked after equally.

The Eastern concept of yin and yang is another important philosophy to consider. Most people are familiar with the classic black-and-white symbol that represents yin and yang, even if they do not know what it stands for. The way in which the two opposites are entwined illustrates the way they work together to achieve ultimate balance. Neither yang nor yin is ever dominant, as each contains an element of the other, held together by an energetic tension. In the quest for balance, yin and yang energies are in constant motion, yin being still, silent and condensed while yang is all that is active, expressive and expansive. This same duality is said to exist in our mind, body and spirit.

Again, whatever our beliefs, we can agree we all have a natural ebb and flow of energy. There are some days when we just wake up tired. We might know the reason for this (a poor night's sleep or a hangover, for example) or we might not. Whatever the reason it is important that we go with the flow. There is no point trying to force ourselves into a highly energetic workout routine when what we really need to do is spend 30 minutes stretching and flexing a tired body.

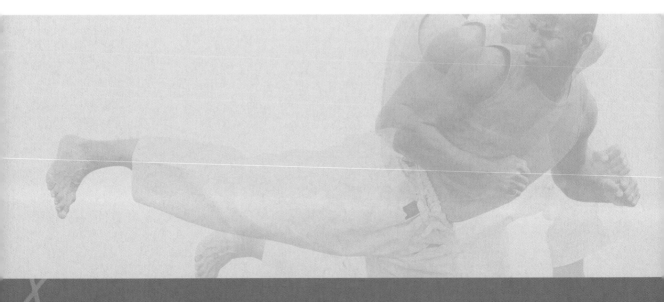

So when should I exercise?

We all have built-in biological rhythms. Researchers who have studied the science of chronobiology – the relationship between your internal body clock, mood and behaviour – say that each of us has unique biological rhythms that have predictable highs and lows. These patterns can not only dictate sleeping and waking patterns but could also mean we are pre-programmed to exercise at a particular time. The diurnal cycle, following the twenty-four-hour light-dark cycle is particularly significant, though some research indicates that a twenty-five-hour cycle might be more normal. What it boils down to is that some of us are more efficient in the morning, others function better at night, and the rest of us are somewhere in between.

For years, the medical profession remained sceptical about the claims that biorhythms can account for many life experiences, but it now is increasingly accepted that they could have a significant influence on our actions and habits. Scientists have carried out studies on the biological rhythms of both humans and animals, and have begun to see that patterns of behaviour have seasonal as well as daily and monthly cycles.

These findings are interesting when viewed alongside the Eastern philosophy of yin and yang. For example we can look at the changing energies within the twenty-four-hour yin/yang cycle. Dawn to mid-morning is considered to be Rising Yang, a perfect time to meditate, exercise or engage in intense mental work. Mid-morning to mid-afternoon is Radiant Yang. This, the warmest part of the day, is when we are usually at our most hospitable and is a good time for meetings, debates and again exercise. Mid- to late-afternoon is Descending Yang. This is often the time of day when many of us feel lethargic. Late afternoon to late evening is Rising Yin. The body is winding down in preparation for sleep therefore it is not an ideal time for exercise. Late evening to dawn is Condensed Yin when deep sleep gives the mind and body an opportunity to refresh and rejuvenate.

So how should we decide when is our right time to exercise? Firstly, although scientists believe that our bodies are best suited to working out in the mornings, it is not necessarily the case for our minds. This is because our muscle temperature and other important physical parameters reach a peak in the afternoon. So the optimum time for a demanding workout is probably between 4pm and 7pm for most people. However the trick is to try to get in tune with your body's natural preferences. It would be great to be able to always exercise during the optimum afternoon time slot, but the truth is most of us are at work then. Spend time experimenting with working out at different times of the day. However much the idea of a 6.30am workout fills you with dread, set the alarm clock and give it a go. You never know, you might surprise yourself.

The Hi-chi workout

BENEFITS

>> WORKS
CARDIOVASCULAR
SYSTEM

>> BURNS CALORIES

>> REDUCES EXCESS FAT

>> IMPROVES
MUSCLE TONE

The Hi-chi Workout combines dynamic kicks from the Korean martial art tae kwon do with plyometric moves. It is designed to be fast moving, explosive and fun! Perfect for burning off calories and working the heart and lungs, helping to improve the cardiovascular system.

Plyometrics is a strength-training method used to develop explosive power. It is an important component of most athletic skills and has been used for many years by athletes to improve their sports performance. However, you don't need to be an athlete to benefit from using plyometrics; it is a great tool for intensifying workouts, consisting of hopping, skipping, jumping and throwing activities designed to improve your power. For instance, a runner who wants to improve her speed could improve her stride length by skipping or hopping. In this context, we can improve kick speed by incorporating dynamic moves into the workout. These high-energy moves not only increase your heart rate and burn calories but also help to improve muscle tone.

There is a low-impact alternative for each plyometric move. If you have had joint problems and/or impact-related injuries (such as shin splints) then you should follow these instead. Start with the warm-up and remember to spend time cooling down and stretching.

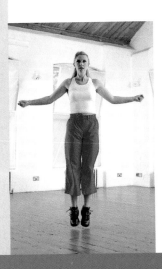

<< **Virtual skipping**
This is basically skipping with an imaginary rope. Start with your feet hip-width apart and your knees soft. Begin to jump your imaginary rope with both feet, landing as softly as possible. Think of your ankles and knees as shock absorbers and allow your body weight sink through.
Low-impact version – As above, but keep your toes on the ground at all times. Lift each heel alternately as though running on the spot. *Continue for 30 seconds.*

Front kicks

1. Start in the fighting stance: stand sideways with your feet shoulder-width apart with your front foot facing forwards and your rear foot slightly outwards. Keep your weight distributed evenly on both legs. Make sure your knees are 'soft' and your weight is on the balls of your feet. With closed fists and bent elbows, keep the arms close to the body. If the left leg is leading then the left bent arm should be in front with the elbow pointing downwards and the fist pointing up. The right arm lies across the chest with the elbow close to the body.

2. Bring your rear leg forward with the knee well bent and the shin vertical.

3. Then extend this leg, letting the upper body move slightly back. The kick is delivered with the ball of the foot with the toes pulled back. Keep elbows and arms firm but relaxed in front of the body. Retract and place the foot down quickly without slamming.

2 sets of 15 on each leg

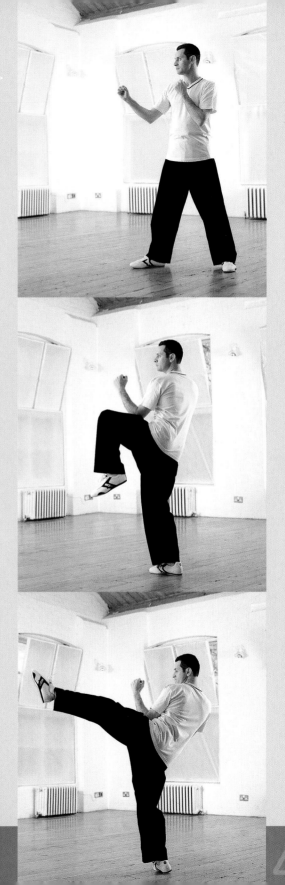

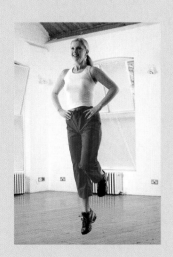

Hopping

Choose a distance of 5 metres, perhaps the length of your hall or longest room. Hop on your right foot to the end, change legs and turn round. Keep your knees and ankles soft and sink into the hop.

Low-impact version – Low-impact skipping as above.

Continue for 30 seconds.

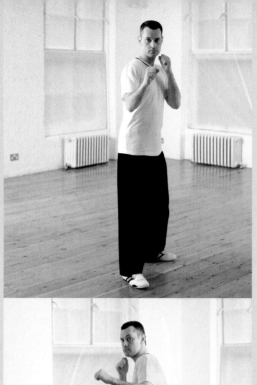

<< **Side kicks**

1. Begin in a fighting stance.
2. Shift your body weight over the rear foot, and raise your front leg up, bending the knee and bringing it as close as possible towards the rear shoulder. Try to bring the foot up to the same height as the knee so that the base of the heel is pointing towards the target.
3. To kick, extend the raised knee so that it follows the heel directly towards the target area.
2 sets of 15 on each leg.

Squat thrusts

1. Place your hands on the floor shoulder-width apart with your fingers facing forwards. Take your legs back until your body is almost in a straight line.
2. Now jump with both feet, bringing your knees in towards your chest. As soon as you land, jump back to the starting position and repeat. Keep your abdominals tight and your bottom low.

Low-impact version

Narrow squats. Stand with your feet shoulder-width apart, knees soft and back straight. Flex at the knees and hips, keeping the back straight. Make sure your knees travel in line with your toes. Squat down until the thighs are roughly parallel to the ground and no further. Straighten up, taking care not to lock the knees at the top of the move. *Continue for 30 seconds.*

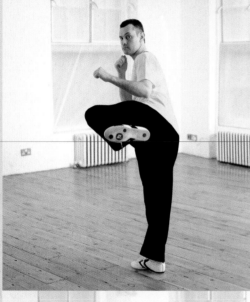

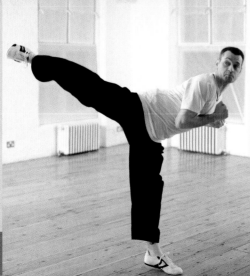

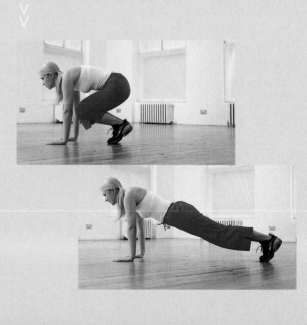

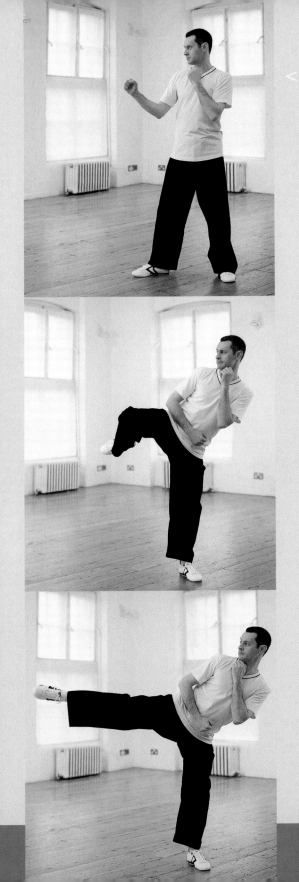

<< **Turning kicks**

1. Begin in the fighting stance. Make sure your supporting foot is turned sideways and that the weight of your body is kept on the bent back leg.

2. Raise the front leg up with the knee well bent.

3. When the knee reaches hip or waist height kick out to the side (either with the instep or the ball of the foot). Use the hips to drive the kick through. Pull the kick back returning to the original stance. Keep your arms and elbows up throughout the kick.

2 sets of 15 on each leg

Squat jumps

1. Start with your feet hip-width apart, arms down by your side.

2. Jump out into a deep squat sinking into your knees as you land. Simultaneously take your arms up and out. Do not bend your knees more than 45 degrees. Jump immediately back to the start position and repeat. Keep your abdominal muscles tight and your back straight.

Low impact version –

Half stars. Start with your feet hip-width apart, arms out slightly bent to the sides. Step the left foot out to the side and take your arms above your head. Return to the centre and repeat with the other side.

Continue for 30 seconds above your head.

Return to the centre and repeat with the other side.

Continue for 30 seconds.

V V

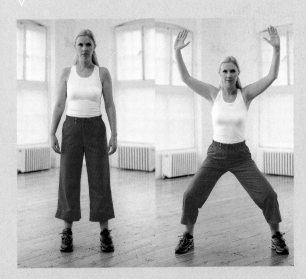

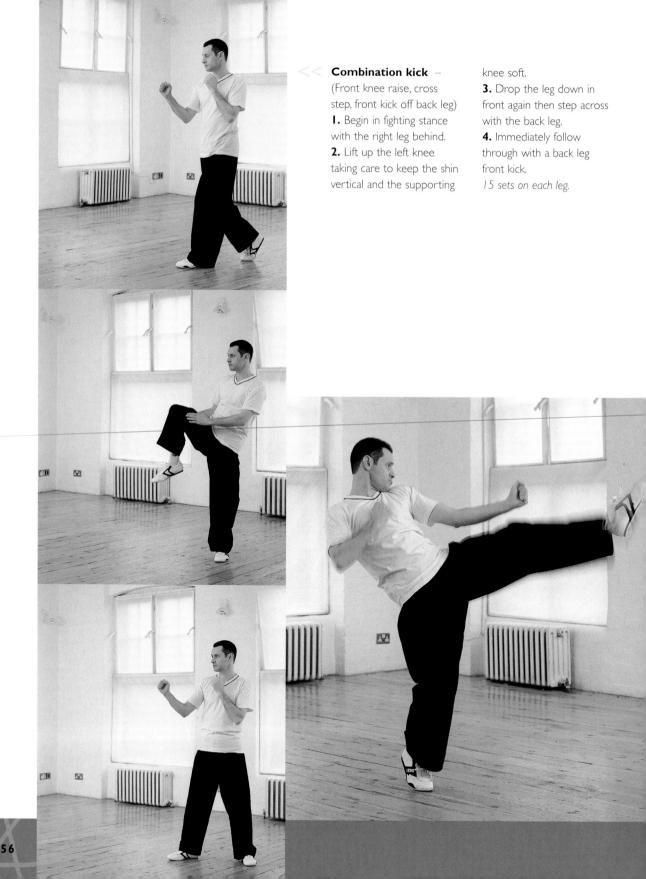

Combination kick –
(Front knee raise, cross step, front kick off back leg)
1. Begin in fighting stance with the right leg behind.
2. Lift up the left knee taking care to keep the shin vertical and the supporting knee soft.
3. Drop the leg down in front again then step across with the back leg.
4. Immediately follow through with a back leg front kick.
15 sets on each leg.

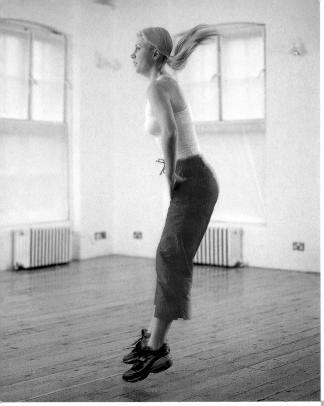

Double leg hops

1. Choose a distance of 3–5 metres. Start with your feet hip-width apart, knees and ankles soft and your hands on your hips.

2. Hop with both feet making sure you sink into your landing. Aim to keep your back straight, abdominal muscles tight and be as light on your feet as possible.

Low impact version –

Single leg lunges. Start with your feet hip-width apart, knees soft and back straight. Lunge back with the left leg, touching your toe behind you on the ground. At the same time take your arms up to shoulder height. Return immediately to the start position and repeat with the other leg.

Continue for 30 seconds.

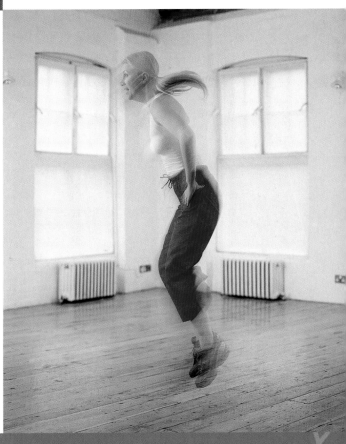

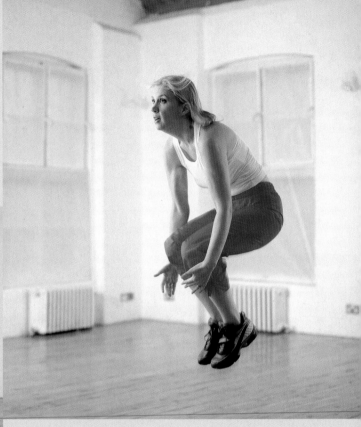

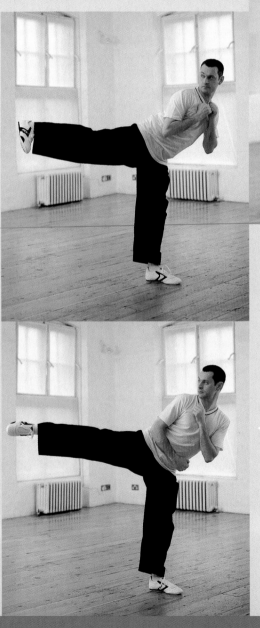

∧
∧

High jumps

Start with your feet hip-width apart, abdominals tight and back straight. Jump up high, trying to tuck both knees into the chest. Land as softly as possible sinking into your knees and ankles. Breathe out as you jump.

Low-impact version

Knee lifts. Standing tall, lift up alternate knees touching opposite knee with opposite hand.
Continue for 15–20 seconds

<< ### Combination kicks –

Side kick to low/mid section followed by turning kick to low/mid section)

1. Begin in fighting stance with the left leg leading. Do a low-section side kick aiming at knee height.

2. Retract the kick back to the start position and follow through with another side kick, this time to the mid section. Return to the original back stance and repeat this time using firstly a low section turning kick followed by a mid section kick.
15 sets on each leg.

Combination kicks –
(Front kick, side kick off front leg followed by turning kick off the back leg.)
1. Start in fighting stance with the right leg behind.
2. Throw a front kick off the back leg, keeping the supporting knee soft and retract it back to its starting position.

3. Then throw a side kick off the front leg dropping it in front, following it immediately through with a back leg turning kick.
15 sets on each leg.

Finish the workout with the Quick all-over stretch from the Healing Hand chapter.

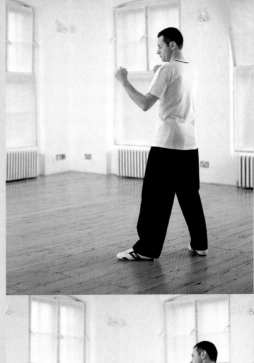

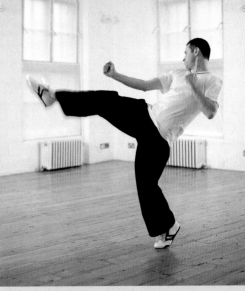

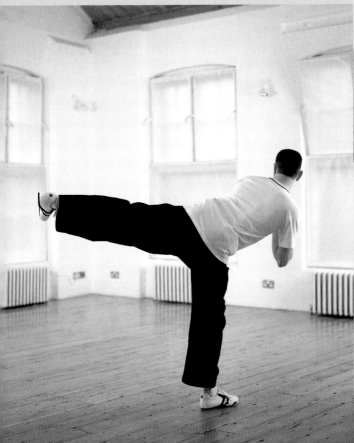

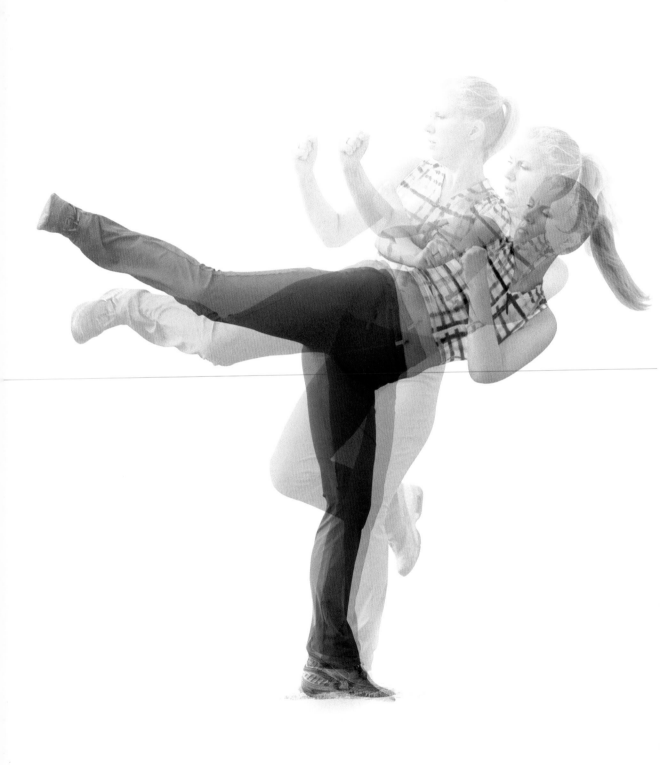

Yin and yang captures the essence of balance, harmony and equality that we should try and have in our everyday lives. Chinese philosophy stresses that for us to be in harmony and balance the whole world around us needs to be in the same harmony and balance. Likewise, if we are not in harmony and balance within ourselves, the whole universe is put out of order. It is vitally important to be aware, to be mentally and physically centred or at least strive towards this. The Law of Balance is a recognition of our own natural limitations. We need to learn to tune into our body's natural awareness and accept this natural law.

THE LAW OF BALANCE >>

So how do we do this? Simply by beginning to realise that some days are good and some are bad. Any change in our equilibrium can throw us off course. If we begin our workout with our mind on something else we are not going to give it our full attention. At least if we realise that we are distracted we can take action. We can either decide to leave our troubles at the door or we can leave the exercise to a different day. Once we accept that for every up day there will naturally be a down day we are on our way to a simpler and more effective life. There is a natural law to everything. It is only human beings that are in such a hurry. In nature the seasons follow each other without haste in the proper sequence. We need to follow our natural cycle – and enjoy it!

The balanced body workout

The Balanced Body workout gives us three separate routines: an upper body a lower-body and an all-over workout. It uses energetic kickboxing punches, kicks and elbows but also incorporates a slower conditioning workout that tones, lengthens and strengthens every muscle group. By giving the body a balanced workout, one or two minutes of fast energetic moves followed by slower more condensed ones, we are learning the art of control and pacing. Throughout this workout we can become aware of how our body moves at different speeds, thereby becoming more in tune with ourselves. You will need a small handweight for the upper-body workout. Pick the workout which suits you in your weekly exercise plan – shut out the world and get involved!

UPPER-BODY WORKOUT >>

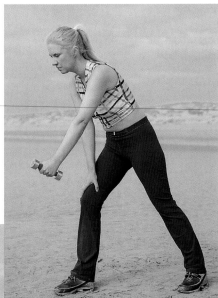

One arm row

1. Stand with your feet hip-width apart holding on to your handweight with your left hand. Step forwards with your right leg, lean forwards and place your right hand and body weight securely on your right thigh. Now, as if to complete a third part of a triangle (foot, foot and handweight), stretch the left hand out backwards. Keep your back straight and your abdominals tight to support your back. Look forward and down.

2. Keeping the wrist straight and leading with the elbow, draw the handweight up to the armpit keeping the arm close to the body. Lower under control until the arm is straight avoiding 'locking out' the elbow joint. Keep this exercise slow and controlled at all times. *Repeat 10–20 times and then change sides. Begin by doing 2 sets on each side and build up to 3.*

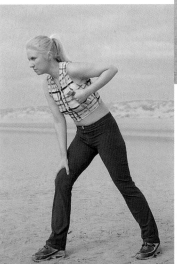

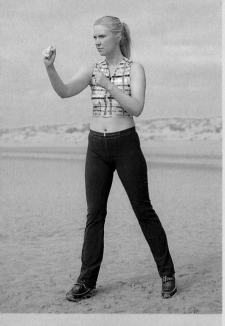

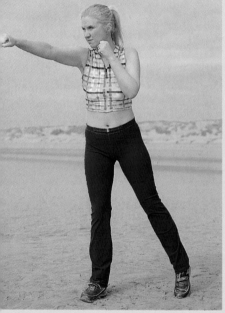

Jab/Cross from fighting stance – <<
1. Start in the fighting stance with your right foot behind. Make sure your weight is evenly distributed between both legs. Keep the knees slightly bent and the back heel slightly off the floor. Keep your arms up with your fists closed, in this stance your left fist should be 5–6 inches (13–15cm) in front of your right.
2. To jab, snap the lead fist out towards the target (a fist width's distance right of centre) taking care not to lock out the elbow. At the same time, turn your shoulders, waist and hips to the right and pivot on the ball of your right foot so your weight moves forwards to your left leg as you punch. Retract your arm and return to the fighting stance. To follow up the jab with a cross, as you retract your lead left hand visualise your target across your left shoulder about 2–3 inches (5–8cm) short of full extension. Punch out with your right fist, lifting your right heel and pivoting to the left. Make sure you use your hips, waist and shoulders to help deliver the punch. Your left leg should be slightly bent, and your weight should shift forwards as you complete the punch. Retract the arm back to fighting stance.
Do a set of 10 with the left leg behind and then swap sides. Remember that this is a dynamic and fast movement.

Skipping – You can skip with >> or without a rope. However a good skipping rope is a fabulous, simple and relatively cheap piece of aerobic equipment. You can either jump with two legs together or just 'skip' over the real or imaginary rope. Don't try and jump too high and keep your knees and ankles soft at all times.
Continue for 30 seconds.

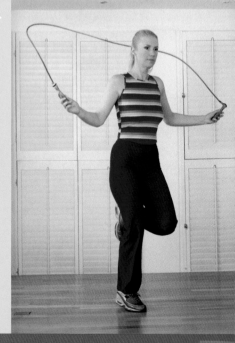

Heel-digs

Place alternate heels in front of you keeping the supporting knee soft. Punch your arms out in front of you with every 'heel-dig'. Remember to keep your back straight and abdominals tight. If you wish to increase the intensity, punch your hands above your head. *Continue for 30 seconds.*

>>

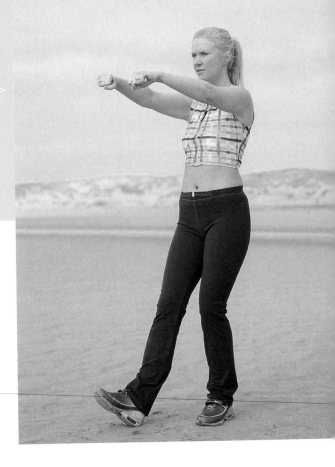

Press-ups

1. Start by kneeling with your hands one and half times shoulder-width apart and your knees directly underneath your hips. Take your knees back so you can cross your ankles and rest your body weight on the fleshy part above your knee-caps. Keep your hands directly underneath the line of your shoulders.

2. Tighten your abdominal muscles making sure you keep your back straight at all times. Flex at the elbows slowly lowering your chin and chest towards the ground. Straighten up making sure you don't lock out your elbows. *Repeat 10–20 times, rest for 30 seconds and repeat again.*

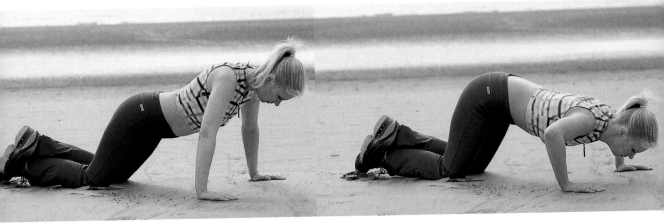

Knee-lifts – Bring one >> knee at a time to the opposite hand. Keep your abdominal muscles tight and your back straight. Do not lean forwards or back and keep the supporting knee slightly bent. To increase the intensity, lift your arms high above your head.
Continue for 30 seconds.

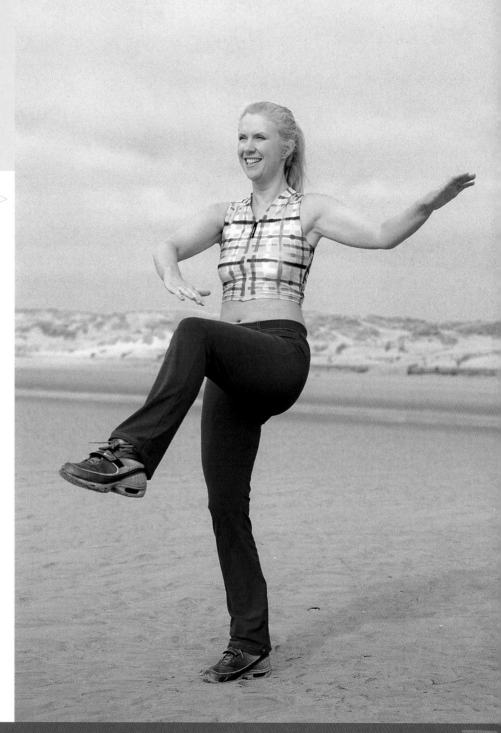

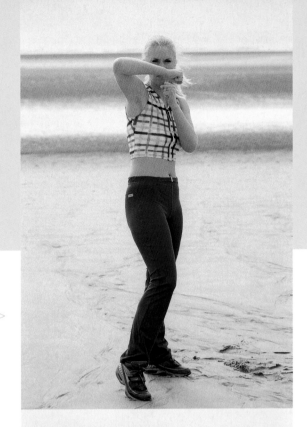

Double hooks >>

1. Start in fighting stance, with your hands up and body weight distributed evenly between both legs.

2. Lift your left arm at the shoulder, so that your left elbow and fist are level. Visualise your fist travelling along a quarter circle, and pivot both feet, making sure your left knee and left hip are following the same path. Stop 2 or 3 inches (5–8cm) short of full extension. Retract your fist, following the same pathway back. Now, by immediately lifting your right arm, follow through with a right hook making sure your right knee and hip follow the same path. Return to fighting stance. Keep this fast moving and powerful.

Do a set of 10–20 and then change leading legs.

Thirty seconds skipping

As before

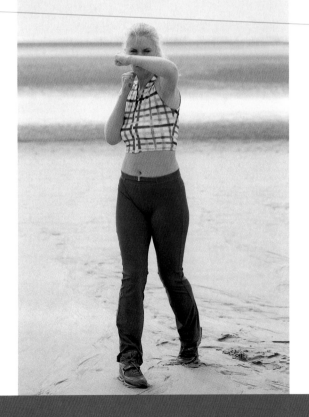

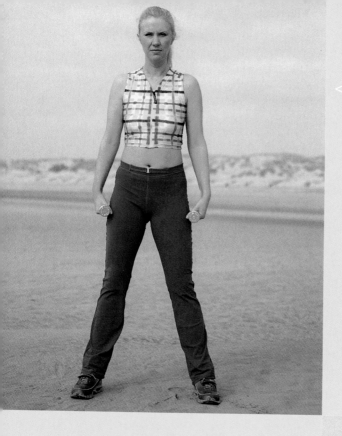

Lateral raises

1. Stand with your feet one and a half times hip-width apart, bottom tucked under and knees slightly soft. Place the handweights to your sides, bend the arms slightly and ensure the wrists are straight.

2. Now, raise the handweights slowly out to the sides of your body leading with the knuckles and keeping the elbows soft.

Do not take your arms higher than shoulder height and try and avoid any unnecessary wrist movement. Lower slowly to the start position.
*Repeat 10–20 times.
Rest for 30 seconds (or do 30 seconds of heel-digs) and then repeat.*

Thirty seconds heel-digs

As before

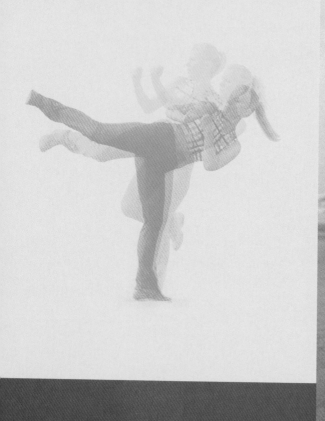

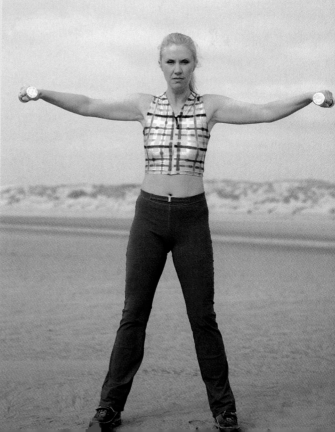

Uppercuts

1. Start from fighting stance but with your hands up in guard position, parallel to your shoulders instead of under your chin. **2.** As you pivot both feet, turn your left knee, left hip, your waist, and your left shoulder to the right and into the punch. At the same time, you want to make sure your right knee is slightly bent so you can give your punch an upward thrust. At the point of impact, your left arm will be 2–3 inches (5–8cm)

short of full extension and your left fist about 12 inches away from your face. Return to the start position and repeat immediately with the right fist following through with the right knee, hip, waist and right shoulder. Return to fighting stance. *Do 10–20 sets and then change leading legs and repeat.*

Thirty seconds knee-lifts

As before

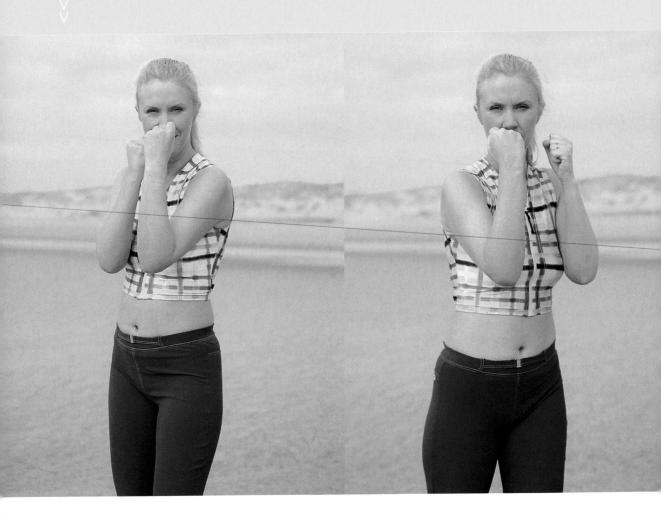

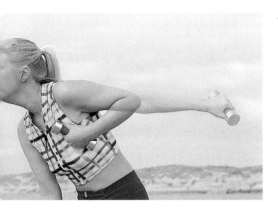

<< **Tricep kickbacks**
Start with your feet hip-width apart and step forwards with your right leg. Lean forwards placing your right hand on your right thigh, keeping your back straight and your abdominal muscles tight. Holding a handweight in your left arm lift your elbow up high (keeping it close to the body), placing the weight by your armpit.

Now, keeping the elbow high and still, straighten the arm as slowly as possible making sure you do not lock out the elbow. Return slowly to the start position. *Repeat 10–20 times. Change sides and repeat. Begin by doing 2 sets on each arm and build up to 3.*

Thirty seconds skipping
As before

Elbows
Start in the fighting stance with your guard up. Raise your front left elbow into a horizontal position, with your hand close to your shoulder. The front elbow strike is thrown just like a hook. However, do not make a fist, because a closed fist will tighten the forearm muscles and make the strike slower. Snap the left shoulder dynamically forwards with the left elbow in the lead. As the elbow moves through the imaginary target, retract the arm back to the start position. To perform the rear elbow, immediately twist the upper body forwards with the right shoulder leading the way.

As the right shoulder >> is coming forwards, raise the right arm into the horizontal position. The right hand will be close to the right shoulder (again, do not make a fist, keep the hand relaxed). As the arm snaps forwards, the elbow extends out and hits the target. Snap elbow back and return to fighting stance.
Do 10–20 sets and then change leading leg and repeat.

Finish off with the Shoulders, neck and back stretch combined with the Back and abdominal stretch or the Quick all-over body stretch from chapter nine.

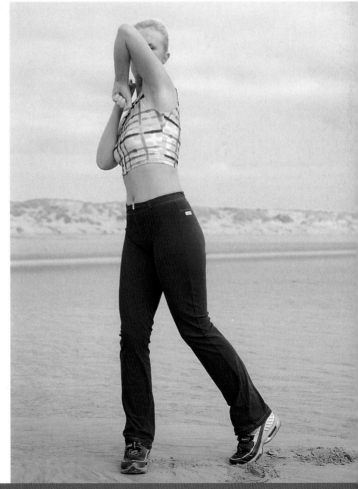

LOWER-BODY WORKOUT

Marching on the spot
Keep your feet softly flexed
and don't slam them down.
Keep your back straight and
abdominal muscles tight.
Pump the arms back and
forth keeping the elbows
slightly bent.
Continue for 30 seconds.

>>

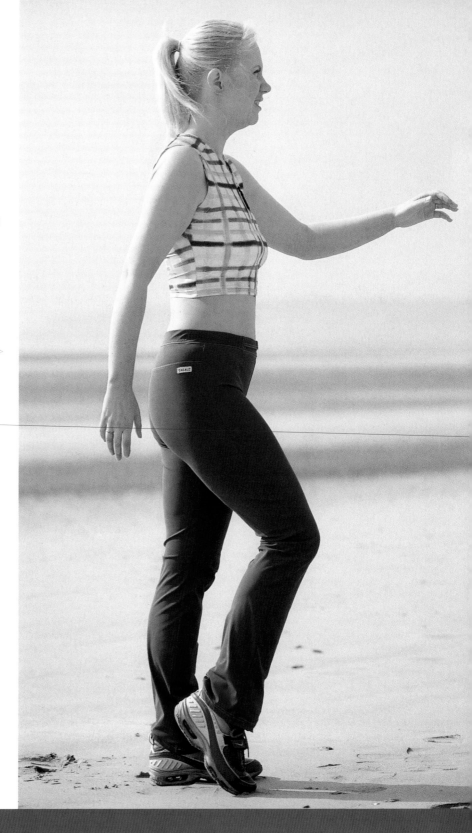

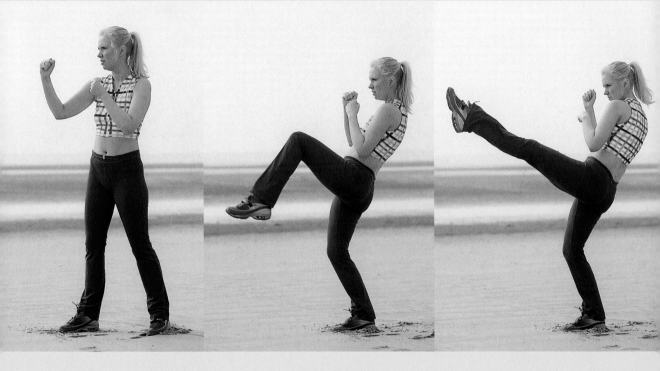

Front kicks

1. Begin in fighting stance with your left leg back. Your feet should be facing forwards, about shoulder-distance apart and your hands up in guard position. Keep about 80 per cent of your body weight on your front right leg, and the rest on the ball of your back leg.

2. Lift your back left leg with the foot pointed into a knee raise and then extend out with the kick making sure not to lock out the knee joint. Snap the foot back into the knee-raise position before dropping the leg back into the original fighting stance. *Do 10–20 and then change legs and repeat.*

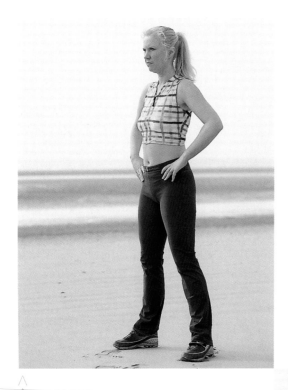

Squats

1. Stand with your feet one and a half times hip-width apart, bottom tucked under, abdominals lifted and back straight.

2. Squat down slowly by flexing at the knees and hips making sure your knees travel in line with your toes. Do not take your bottom any lower than the line of your knees and keep your heels firmly on the ground. Straighten up taking care not to lock out your knee joints. *Do 10–20 squats, rest for 30 seconds (or do 30 seconds of backward lunges) and then repeat once more.*

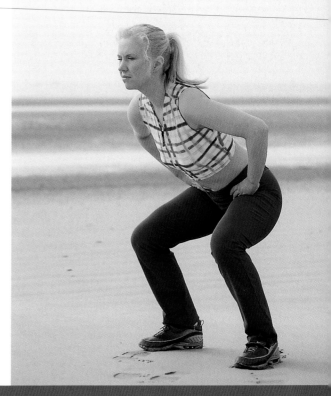

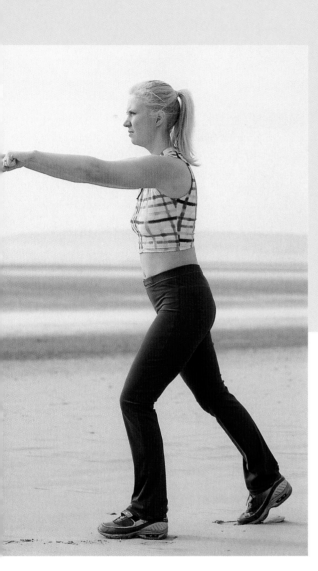

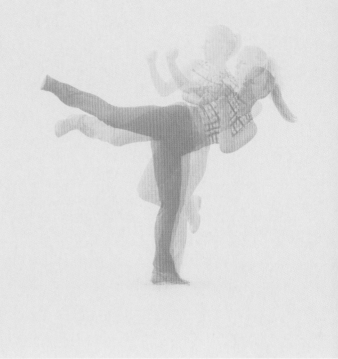

<<

Backwards lunge –
Start with your feet hip-width apart, hands by your side. Lunge back with alternate legs whilst simultaneously punching your arms up in front of you. Make sure it is only the ball of the lunging foot that is on the ground and keep your abdominals tight.
Continue for 30 seconds

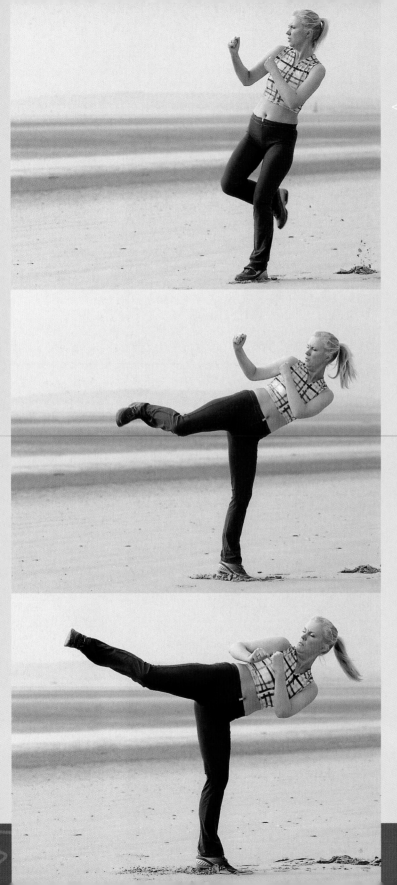

<< **Side kicks**

1. Start in fighting stance with your left leg behind and your guard up. Take 80 per cent of your body weight on to your slightly bent back leg. The remainder of your body weight should be concentrated on the ball of your front right foot so you are ready to move.

2. In one movement, lift your right heel and knee as high as you comfortably can. However high that is, it is important that your right heel and knee are on the same level. As you kick out, allow the hip to roll over or turn into the kick.

3. The kick thrusts out in a straight line with the striking area being the heel of the foot. Make sure your heel is slightly higher than your toes to help land the kick. Snap the leg back into the fold as quickly as possible and set in down in your original fighting stance.

Do 10–20 kicks and then change leading leg and repeat.

Marching on spot
As before
Continue for 30 seconds.

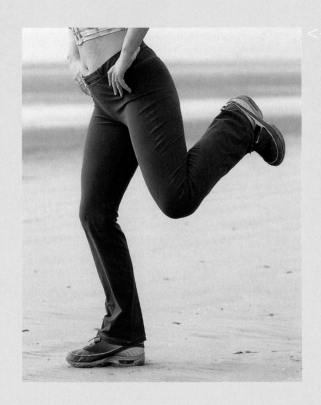

<< **Leg curls**

Start with your legs one and a half times hip-width apart, knees slightly soft and body upright. Slowly, by transferring your supporting body weight on to the opposite leg, squeeze one heel slowly towards your bottom. Keep your supporting knee soft. Return the leg as slowly as possible to the starting position. Change legs and repeat. *Do 40–50 leg curls, rest for 30 seconds (or lunge back for 30 seconds) and then repeat once more.*

Backwards lunge

As before
Continue for 30 seconds.

Lunges

1. Start with your feet hip-width apart and toes facing forwards.
2. Step directly forwards with the right leg so that both knees bend to a right angle as the body is lowered. Keep your body upright with your feet hip-distance apart. Look forwards and slightly down. Drive back with the forward right leg and then repeat on the left.
Do 10–20 lunges, march for 30 seconds and repeat.

Marching on spot

As before
Continue for 30 seconds.

∨
∨

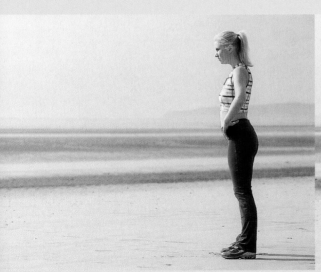

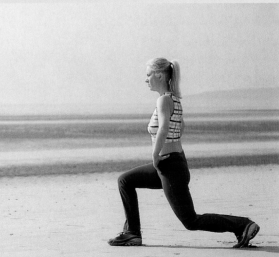

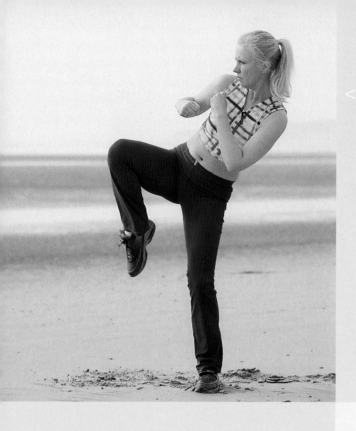

<< **Roundhouse kicks**

1. Begin in fighting stance with your left leg behind and your guard up. Shift about 80 per cent of your body weight on to your back leg keeping the knee slightly bent. The remainder of the weight should be on the ball of the front foot, so again you are ready to move. As you lift the front kicking leg, let the body turn sideways or pivot back as you point the knee towards the target.

2. With the kicking foot in a hard point, quickly snap the kick out visualising hitting the target with the lower part of the shin. Snap the leg back into the fold and set it back down in your original stance.
Do 10–20 kicks and then change leading leg and repeat.

Backwards lunges
As before
Continue for 30 seconds.

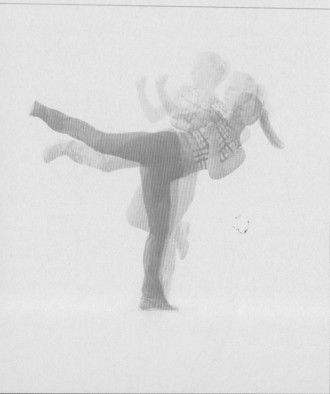

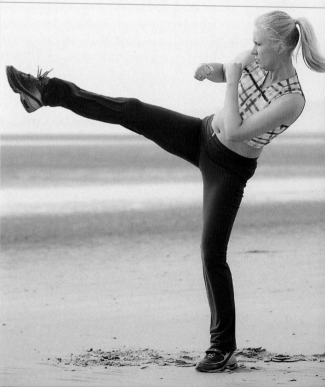

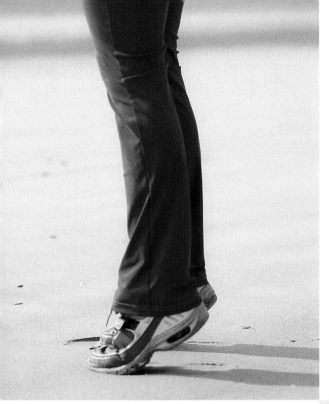

<< **Calf raises**
Standing with your feet hip-width apart and your knees slightly soft. Raise yourself up on to your toes keeping your knees slightly bent throughout. Keep your weight distributed evenly over the balls of your feet and keep the move slow and controlled. If you find yourself wobbling, start by holding on to a chair or nearby wall. Think of lifting up and not tilting forwards or back. Return as slowly as possible to the ground and repeat.
Do 40–50 calf raises.

Marching on spot
As before
Continue for 30 seconds.

Curtsy squats
1. Stand with your feet wider than your shoulders and place your hands on your hips. Hold your abdominals tight to support your back and to aid balance. Slowly cross your left leg bend the right in a curtsy, bending the knees and squeezing your butt. With left knee behind right buttock, press down on the left toes and shift your weight on to right buttock (press right hip slightly upwards).

2. Contract bottom and thighs and pulse down twice, then raise yourself and bring legs back to the starting position.
Do 10 controlled curtsies on the left leg, then switch legs and repeat.

Finish off with either the Quick all-over stretch or the Hips and buttocks stretch combined with the Legs and knees stretch.

>>

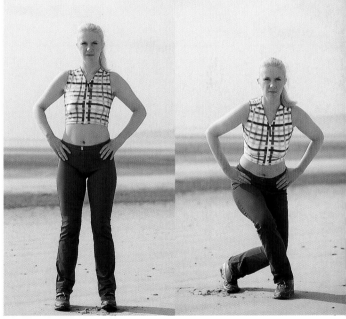

WHOLE-BODY WORKOUT

Jab, cross and front kick
1. Start in the fighting stance with right leg behind and guard up. Throw a jab with your lead left hand.
2. Immediately follow up with a right-handed cross.
3. As you retract the cross, throw a right leg front kick. Return to fighting stance. *Repeat 10–20 times. Change leading legs and repeat.*

∨ ∨

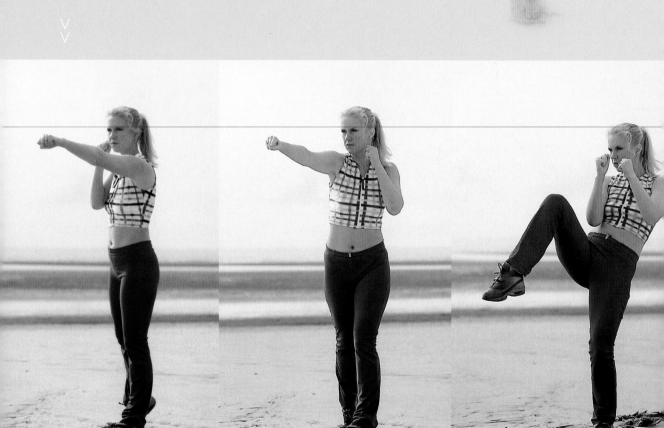

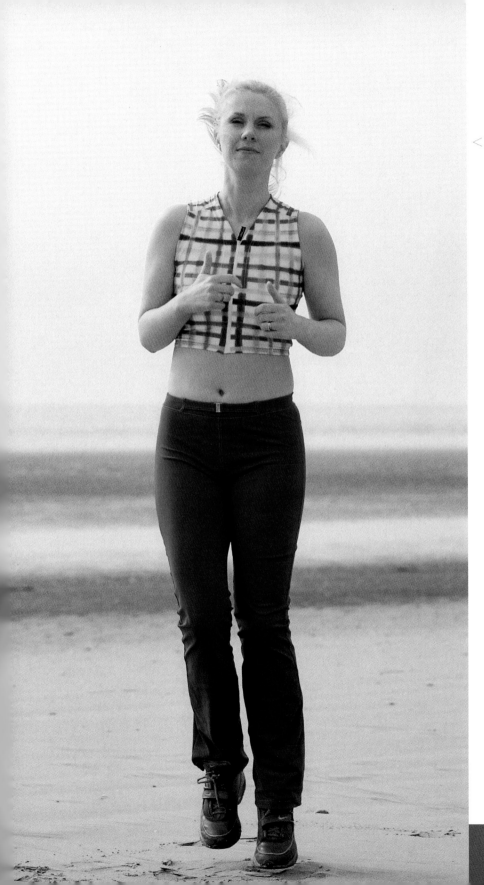

<< **Jogging**
Begin jogging on the spot keeping your knee and ankle joints soft. Keep your elbows softly flexed and gently pump backwards and forwards. If you have enough room jog around taking care to keep your footfall as soft as possible.
Continue for 30 seconds.

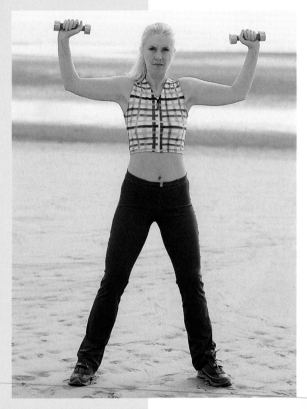

<<

Squats and pec deck

1. Stand with your feet one and a half times hip-width apart, bottom tucked under and shoulders back and down. Lift up your arms at right angles trying to get your elbows parallel to the line of your chest.

2. As you squat down squeeze your forearms together keeping the elbows high. Do not squat any lower than the line of your knees and make sure your knees travel in line with your toes. Return to the start position.
Repeat 10–20 times. Rest for 30 seconds (or do 30 seconds of half stars) and then repeat again.

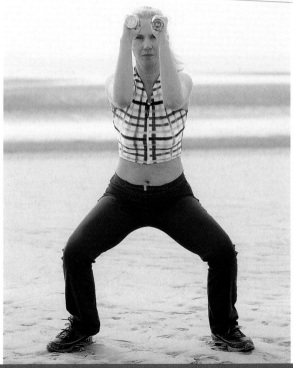

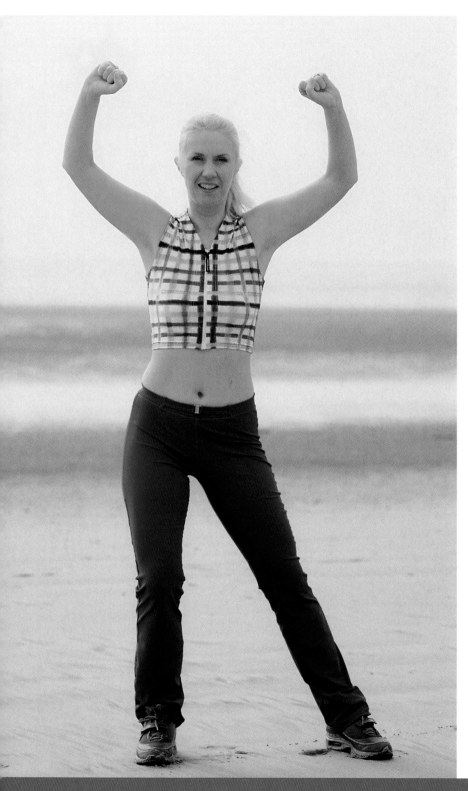

Half stars

Stand with your feet hip-width apart and arms by your side. Step out with the left leg simultaneously taking both arms above your head. Remember to keep both your knees and elbows soft and your back straight. Take leg back to central starting position, change legs and take arms above head again. Keep repeating.
Continue for 30 seconds.

Hook, hook and side kick

1. Begin in fighting stance with your right leg behind and your guard up.

2. Throw a double hook, first with the left and then follow immediately through with a right.

3. As you finish the second hook, lift up your front left leg bringing your heel and knee as high as comfortable and kick out with a side kick. Return to fighting stance. *Repeat 10–20 times. Change leading leg and repeat*

Jogging

As before
Continue for 30 seconds.

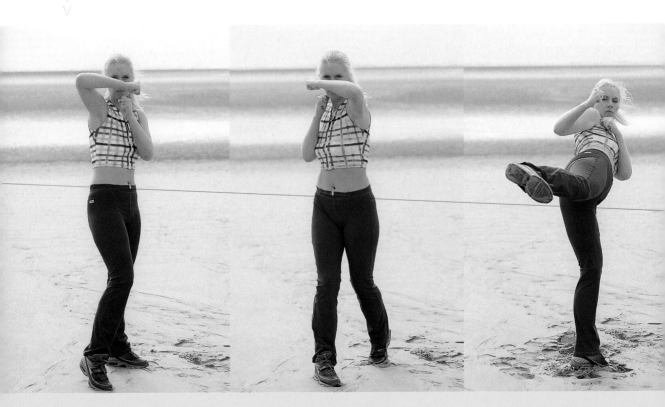

Lunges and lateral raises

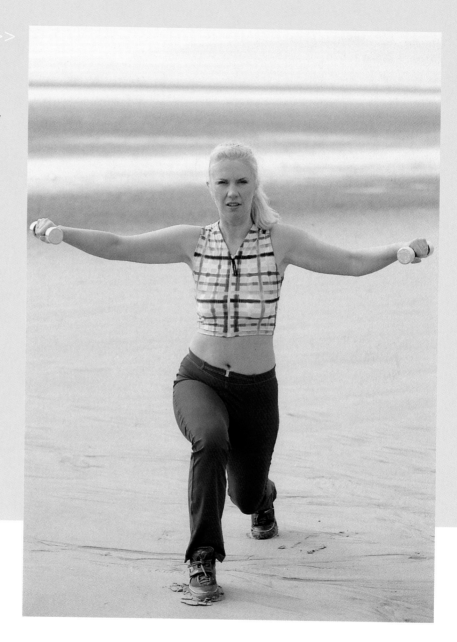

Start with your feet hip-width apart and toes facing forwards. Arms are by your sides with the elbows slightly bent. Step forwards with the right leg so that both knees bend to a right angle as the body is lowered. At the same time raise both arms up to shoulder height keeping the palms facing down. Keep your body upright with your feet hip-distance apart. As you drive back with the leading leg, lower the arms back to your side. Repeat on the other leg, again lifting the arms to shoulder height.
Repeat 10–20 times, rest for 30 seconds (or do 30 seconds of half stars) and repeat.

Half stars

As before
Continue for 30 seconds.

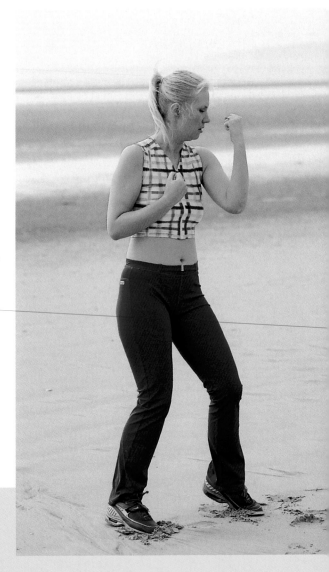

Upper cut, upper cut and knee

1. Start in fighting stance with the right leg behind and your guard up.

2. Throw a left-hand upper cut following immediately through with a right-hand one. Pivot with your feet and use your knees, hips, waist and shoulders to get under the punches.

3. As you finish the second punch shift your weight on to your back supporting leg, then shoot the front knee up and deliver a strike with the bone just above the kneecap. Return to fighting stance.
Repeat 10–20 times.
Change leg and repeat.

Finish off with the Quick all-over stretch.

>>

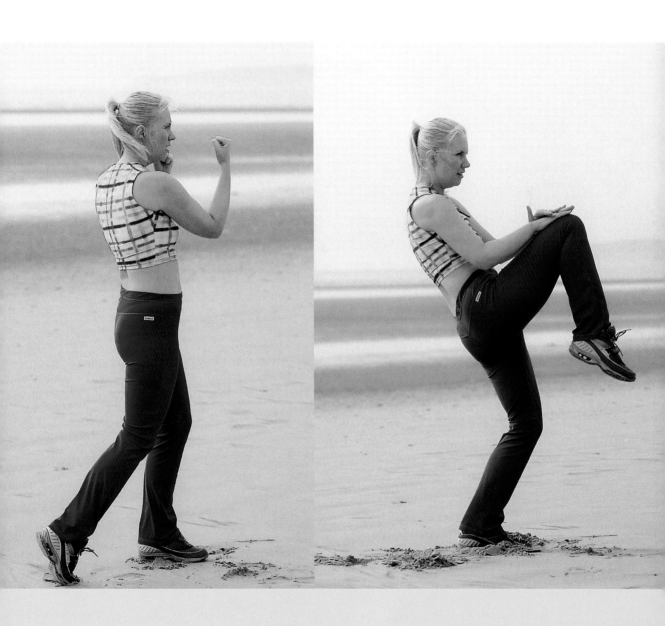

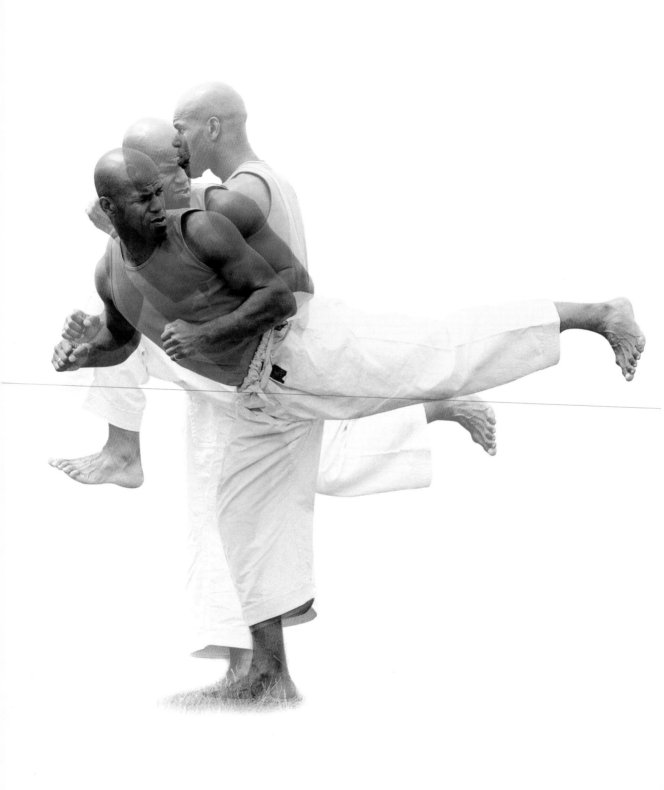

If you are a novice to meditation and sit down with your eyes shut, you will quickly become aware of the stimuli that are normally on the threshold of your conscious thought.: the buzzing of a fly, the passing traffic, aches and pains and above all, the constant stream of thoughts that you are trying to block out. It is incredibly hard to focus your attention, and an art in itself to train the mind to rid itself of inward distractions. A trained athlete learns to tune his or her attention to the here and now. Thoughts still come and go, but attention is focused on the present moment.

THE MIND MAZE >>

We can all gain enormous benefits from learning to concentrate during workouts. Gyms and aerobic classes are full of people half-heartedly going through the motions, hence the dropout rate when boredom sets in and goals are not achieved. In order to gain we need to give.

Think back. Has there ever been a time when you suddenly realised that you are virtually home, but have no recollection of the journey? Or during a conversation it occurs to you that you haven't heard a word anyone has said? Moments like these show how the human mind can work on differing levels. Your eyes and ears may be open, but your focus and attention are captured by thought. This attention can go either way; outwards to a bustling world, or inwards to thoughts.

THE MIND MAZE WORKOUT

The Mind Maze workout consists of exercises based on karate-do. It is designed to work the muscles for strength and endurance. This does not mean, however, that you are going to bulk up like a body builder. Only a hard daily workout with heavy weights can produce this effect. Instead, this workout is designed to create strong and enduring muscles and give you a long and lean all-over muscle tone.

During this workout, try to slow down and concentrate on one aspect alone – the workout itself. This technique can be applied to any of the workout routines in this book. Treat the workout as an active meditation. Turn off the 'phone, lock the door and hide any watches or clocks. If you wish to set yourself a time limit or reminder, then set an alarm clock (on low). Begin by spending your warm-up actively shutting out the hustle and bustle of random thoughts. Work through a checklist of all the things you are NOT going to think about, mentally 'storing' them away for later. Now begin to focus on just how your body is moving and feeling on this particular occasion.

There will be days, despite our best efforts, when this type of required focus is impossible. This does not mean that you should abandon the workout – sometimes working through these moods can help. As long as we realise that, as with life, for every 'up' we should expect a 'down' (and taking into account the 'two steps forwards and one step back' law of life) then we can begin to see that things, in this case our workout results, tend to balance themselves out in the end.

MENTAL BALANCE

This exercise demonstrates how your mental state can affect your inner and outer balance.

The next time you are feeling happy and relaxed, stand up and balance on one leg. If you find this incredibly easy, try it with your eyes closed. Make a mental note of how you feel.

Then try the same exercise when you are feeling angry, annoyed, upset or unsettled. One of two things will happen: if you are holding on to and thinking about your particular 'upset', you will lose your balance easily. If you are meditating on your balance, then you will lose your problem. Physical balance and being upset, like oil and water, just don't mix.

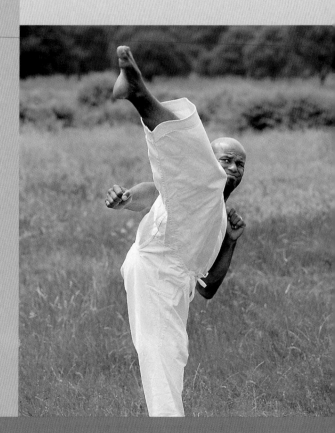

VISUALISATION

Visualisation is a powerful tool for achieving faster and better workout results. By mentally 'feeling' and 'seeing' in your mind's eye the working muscles rise and fall, by imagining how you wish that particular body part to look, you will become much more in tune with your body. This type of training can be used during warm-up, workout and stretching. So how do you visualise? Let's use stretching as an example. Begin by 'seeing' the muscle you are stretching. Hold this visual image in your mind, where that particular muscle begins, and where it goes. This helps to establish a brain-muscle connection, training the muscle group by honing the neurological relationships. As you begin to stretch, visualise the muscle lengthening. Another part of 'tuning in' can be the use of touch. A lot of fitness trainers use 'touch training' in order to optimise their clients' workout benefits. Since the majority of us will be working alone this method in its entirety cannot help us but we can use the simple principle by using the power of our own touch to help us focus fully on the muscle groups we are working.

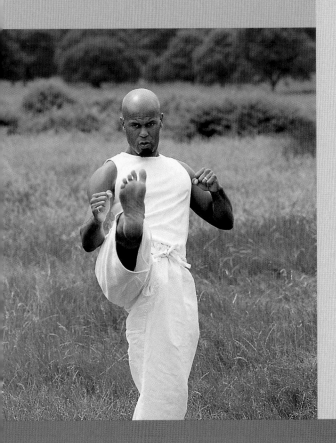

GETTING FOCUSED

Make sure you have plenty of time and a private uninterrupted space to do your workout. A mirror, preferably full length, will help to focus your attention on what you are doing. To begin, talk through the exercise you are doing, for example:

ANKLE JOINT STRETCHES

'I am going to mobilise and flex all the muscles surrounding my ankle joints.'

Touch the muscles around the ankle area so you can mentally pinpoint where you are about to work. Now begin to visualise the ankle joint muscles. Keeping this in mind, begin by getting yourself into the correct position by saying: 'I am going to stand with my feet hip-width apart, my body weight is evenly distributed between both feet.' As you say or think this stand with your feet hip-width apart, and 'feel' yourself actively grounding into the floor. Shift your weight from side to side and then come back to even weight on both feet. Feel your toes spread and make even contact with the floor. 'I am going to let my arms hang loosely by my side' – now think of your shoulders relaxing but not rounding, fingers reaching down along the side of your body stretching out towards the ground. Mentally 'see' energy escaping from your finger tips, boring into the floor by your feet.

Carry on like this throughout the workout aiming to feel focused and centred during its entirety. As with all of the workouts make sure you have a good warm-up and cool-down stretch.

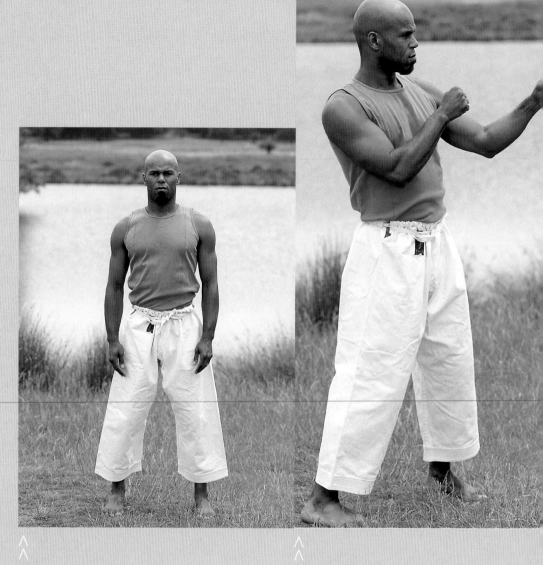

Basic stance
Stand as tall as possible,
keep your hands relaxed
letting them hang loosely by
your sides. Your feet should
be parallel and shoulder-
width apart. Keep your
knees soft. Body weight
should be evenly distributed
between both feet.

Fighting stance
Stand with your feet hip-
width apart, with your left
or right foot forwards and
your hands up in a defensive
posture, with fists loosely
clenched. Keep your knees
slightly bent and concentrate
on keeping pressure through
the balls of the feet.

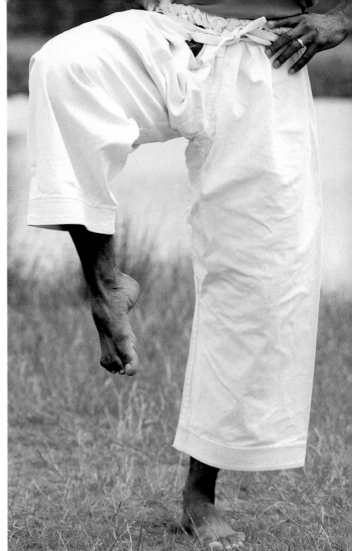

Circling the toes

Start in the basic stance. Raise the big toe of both feet as high as you can off the floor, lifting the toes. At the same time, grip the floor with all the other toes imagining them to be the suction cups of an octopus. Now reverse the motion, raising the four small toes of both feet as high as you can off the floor, curling them upwards. At the same time, grip the floor firmly with the big toes. *Repeat 20 times on each foot.*

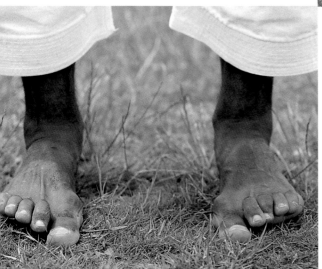

Ankle rotations

Start in the basic stance. Keeping the supporting knee soft and maintaining your balance, lift one heel to hip-height and rotate it inwards whilst keeping the toes firmly pressed into the floor. *Repeat 10 times on each ankle.*

Ankle stretches

1. Start off in basic stance. Begin by raising the inner parts of both feet off the floor. At the same time, press the outer edge of both feet firmly into the floor. Now reverse the motion, raise the outer edge of both feet whilst pressing the inner part firmly into the floor.
Repeat 10 times on each foot.
2. Now repeat the above but this time use the toes of the left and right foot in reverse motion to each other.
3. Lift your heels so you are standing on your toes.
4. Now draw the hips backwards, at the same time slamming your heels down against the foot, letting your toes lift up high. This exercise is designed to stretch the calf muscles and Achilles tendon.
Repeat 20 times.

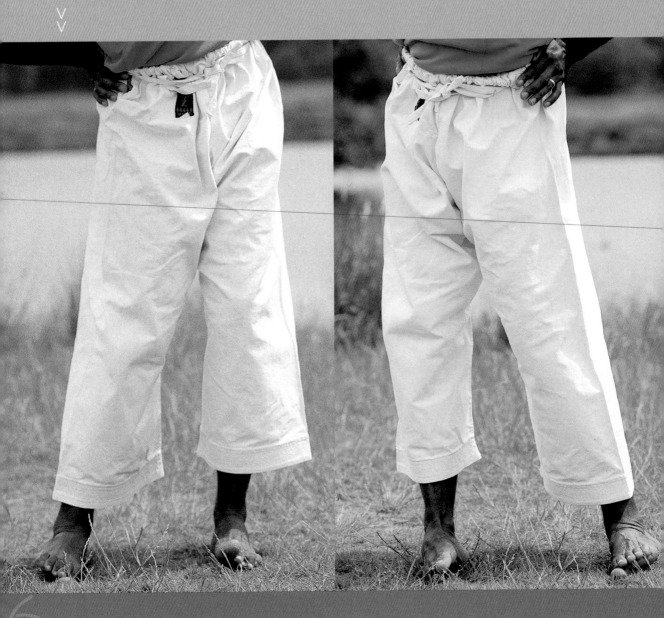

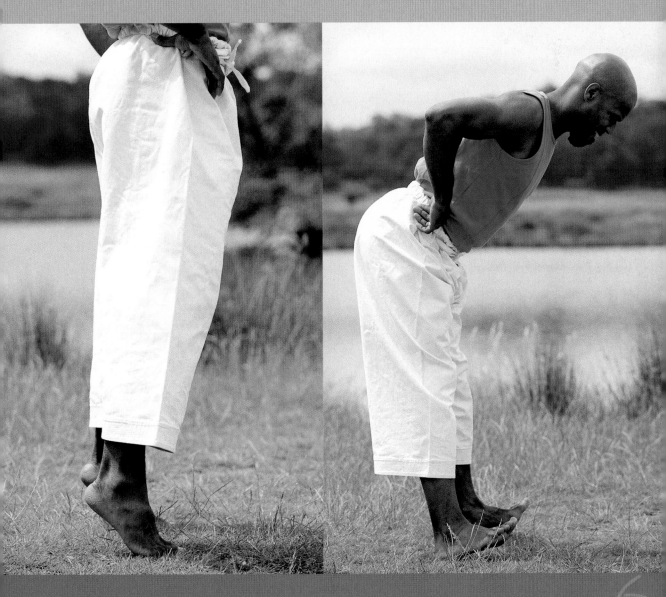

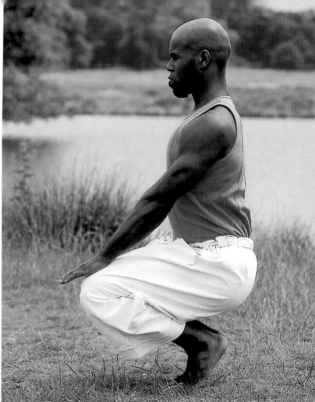

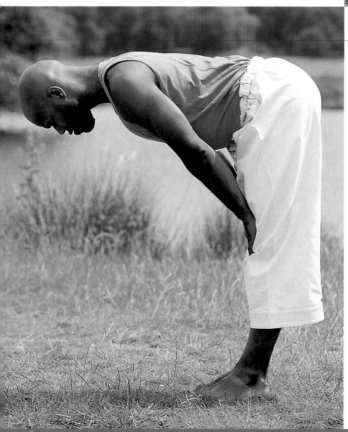

Knee exercises

1. Stand with your feet together. Begin by pressing firmly against both knees with both hands.
2. Squat down slowly keeping the back straight and then return to a standing position.
Repeat 10 times.
3. Now stand with both heels together with your feet at right angles to each other. Starting with your knees together, squat down gradually rotating the knees outwards. From the full squat position with the knees wide apart, stand up rotating them inwards.
Repeat 10 times.

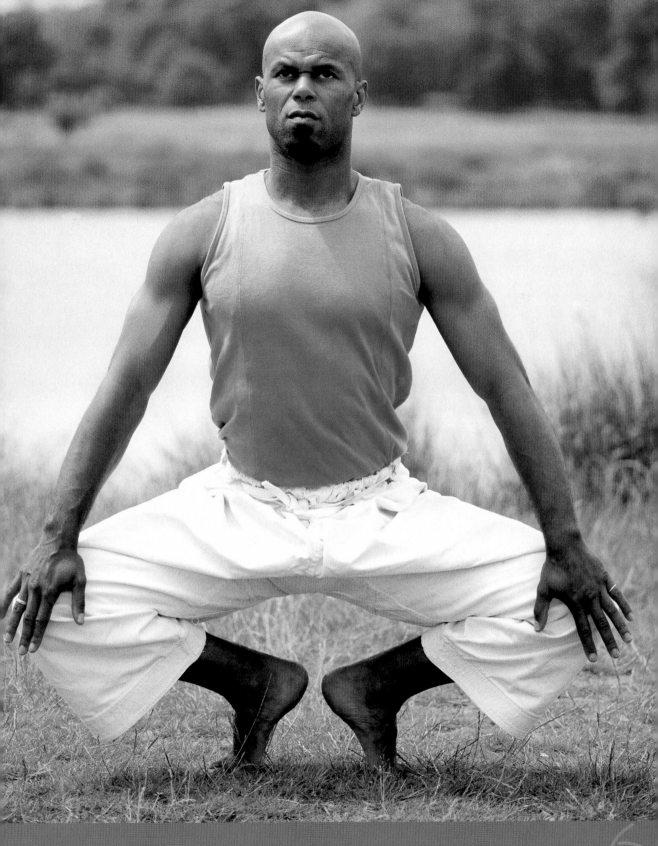

Ankle and pelvic joint exercises

1. Stand in the horse stance, with your feet twice shoulder-width apart. Keeping your feet firmly on the floor, toes pointed outwards, squat down on the right leg keeping the left leg straight, stretching the instep and knee joint. *Alternate 5 times on each side.*

Repeat with the toes pointing forwards to stretch the side of the knee and the pelvic joints.

2. Next, stand with your feet twice shoulder-width apart, go down into a full squat position whilst keeping the left leg straight and raising the toes. This stretches the back of the thigh muscle (hamstring) and your calf muscles. Exhale as you go into the stretch.

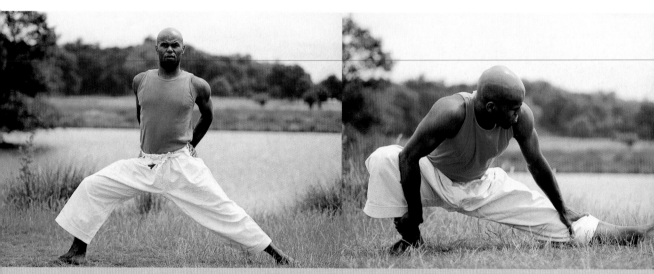

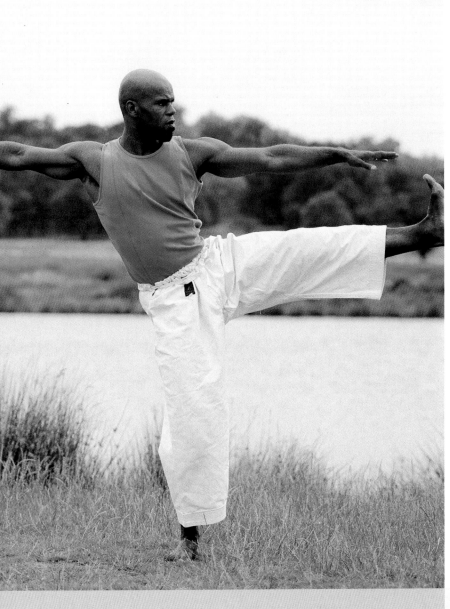

<<

Leg raises

1. Start in the basic stance with arms raised to shoulder height. Keeping your legs fully extended alternately lift them to the corresponding hand. *Do 10 on each leg.*

2. Repeat with your arms extended diagonally and finally with your arms out to the side.

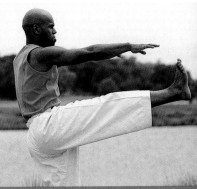

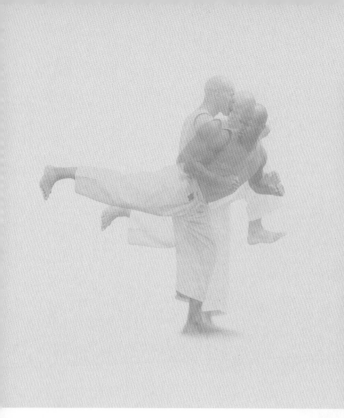

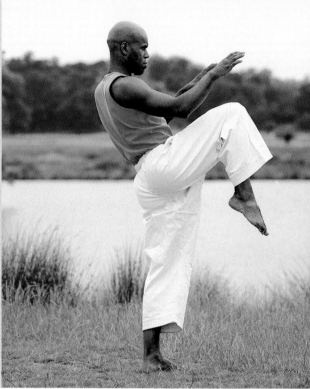

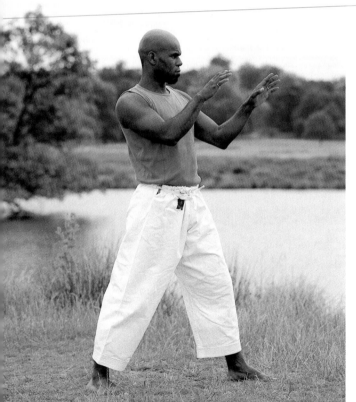

<<

Knee raises

1. Start in the fighting stance with your left leg leading .

2. Lift the right knee up to chest height and drive the hips forwards.

Make sure this exercise is performed vigorously! Return to the fighting stance.

Repeat 10 times. Change leading leg and repeat.

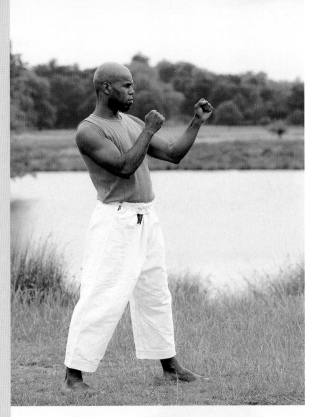

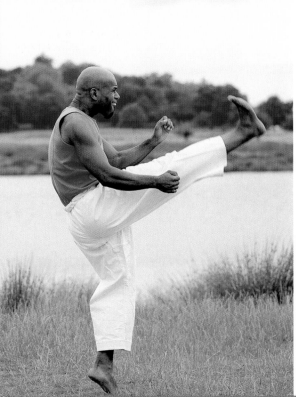

Leg swings
1. Start in the fighting stance with your left leg leading.
2. Swing the extended right leg up to shoulder height trying to keep the leg as straight as possible. Repeat 10 times on each leg. These can be combined with the knee raises as an endurance exercise.
Repeat up to 50 times on each side.

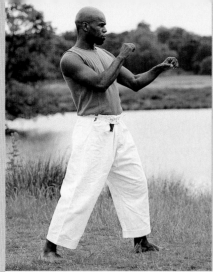

Front kicks

1. Start in the basic stance.

2. Raise the right knee and kick forwards at groin level, focusing on the ball of the foot.

3. Snap the kick back and change legs. Keep the supporting leg soft and arms in a defensive position. Begin by kicking slowly and then gradually increase your speed. As with all the kicks, begin by kicking at an imaginary low target (start as low as knee height) and then slowly try to kick higher. Concentrate first on kicking correctly, powerfully and quickly at the height that is most comfortable for you.

Start with 30 kicks on each leg. For a strength and endurance workout slowly build up to 100 kicks on each leg.

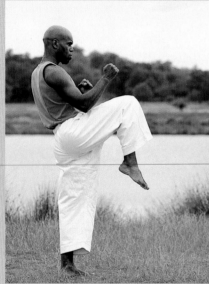

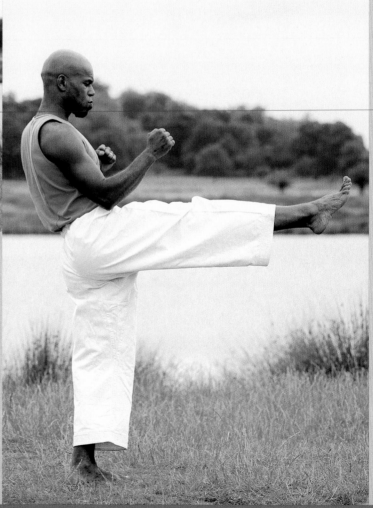

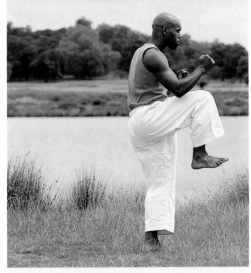

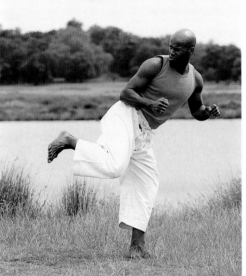

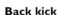

Back kick
1. Start in the basic stance. Raise the knee and ankle up to hip level and tense the muscles of the side.
2. Flexing your ankle and focusing on your instep, kick to the side.
3. Extend through your leg and rotate through your hips.
Do 30 kicks on each leg. Build up to 100 kicks for a strength and endurance workout.

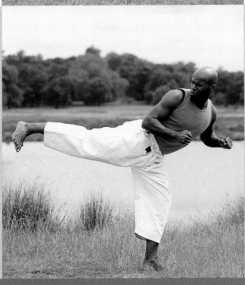

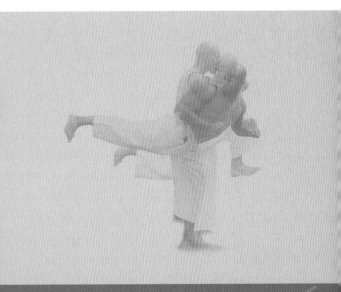

The following exercises were adapted from a selection originally developed by Miyagi Chojun Sensai, founder of Goju Ryu Karate-do.

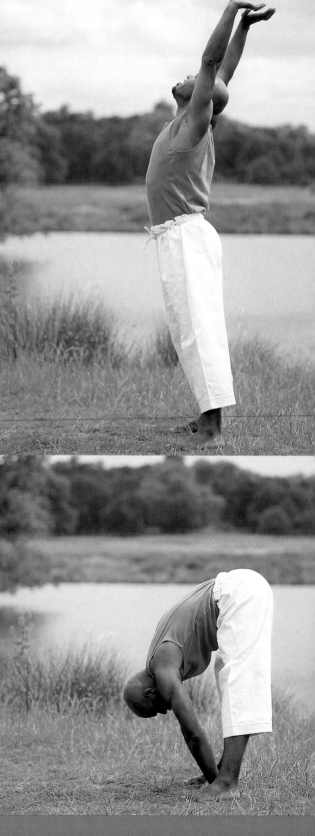

Stretching and bending

1. Start in the basic stance and raise your arms above your head. Slowly bend the upper body forwards from the waist and touch the floor with both hands. Breathe out slowly as you stretch.
Repeat three times.

2. Now stretch the upper body up and backwards.
Repeat 10 times.

3. Stand with your feet wide apart. Bend the upper body forwards diagonally from the waist. Bring your chest down to your knee and touch the floor with both hands. Stretch the hands up and backwards along with the upper body.
Repeat 3 times.

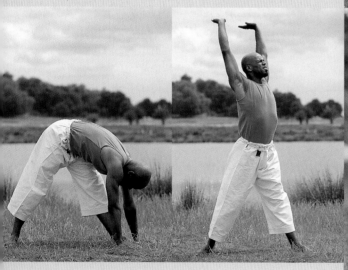

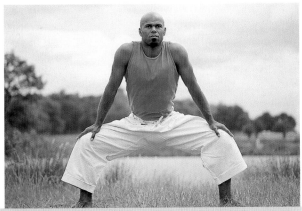

Exercises for the shoulder joint

1. Assume a wide squat stance, placing your hands on your knees.

2. Bend forwards and gently push the right shoulder diagonally across. Then follow through with the left. *Repeat 5 times with each shoulder.*

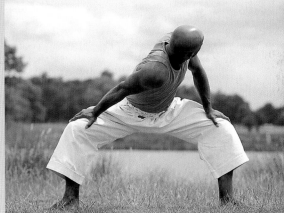

Thrusting the open hands high overhead

1. Start in a high wide stance. Keep one hand at your side and the other on your thigh.

2. Inhale deeply through the nose, then drop into a wide squat position whilst thrusting the open hand high overhead and exhaling explosively. Return to your start position.

Repeat 10 times on each hand. Build up to 50 repetitions with each hand for strength and endurance work.

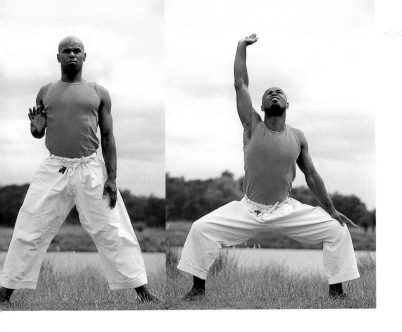

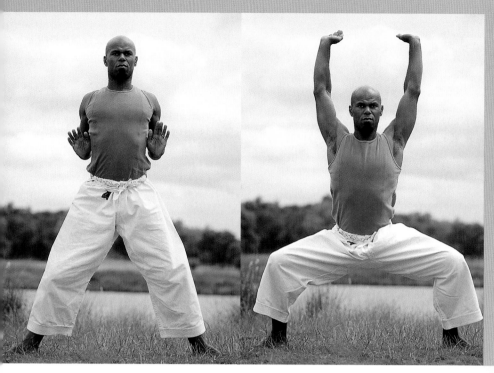

Thrusting both hands high overhead

1. Start in a wide squat position, but this time keep both hands by your sides.

2. Now drop your hips and at the same time thrust both hands high overhead, extending the arms straight up in line with the ears. Exhale explosively through the mouth as you thrust. Stand up again by tightening your butt muscles and straightening through the legs, slowly returning your arms to your sides.

Repeat 10 times building up to 50 repetitions for a strength and endurance workout.

<<

>>

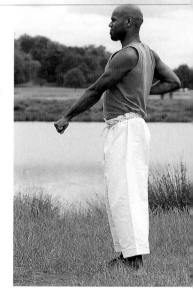

Punches

1. Start in the basic stance with both fists at your sides.

2. Thrust your right fist forwards, aiming at the solar plexus. As you do this twist the right fist inwards whilst delivering the punch. Focus all your power in the first two knuckles at the moment the elbow becomes straight.

Simultaneously draw the left fist to your side, tightening the muscles of the back, wrist, elbow, joints of knees, shoulders, ankles and the soles of the feet at the moment the elbow is straightened.

Repeat at upper (face) level 30 times with each fist.

Repeat at lower (groin) level 30 times with each fist.

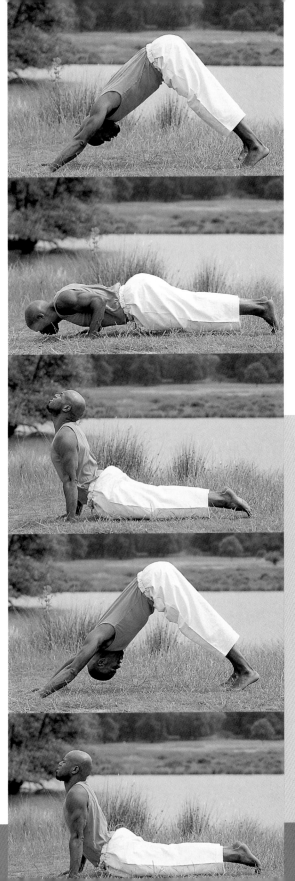

<<

Push-ups (cat style)

This exercise develops neck, hip and forearm muscle. The movement imitates a cat stretching as it wakes up, so think 'graceful and flowing'.

1. Start in the basic stance with your feet parallel and shoulder-width apart, arms hanging relaxed by your sides. Bend forwards from the waist and place both hands on the floor. Keep the soles of your feet firmly on the floor and tuck your chin in whilst straightening your back, aiming to form a pyramid shape.

2. Lower the body into normal push-up position, supporting your body weight with bent arms. Now lift your chin, arching your neck backwards whilst exhaling through the mouth. Look left and right whilst continuing to exhale, then look down towards the floor.

3. Draw the hips backwards, straightening the arms to return to the original pyramid shape and inhale slowly through the nose.

4. Finish by dropping the hips down to the floor quickly. Straighten the arms and arch the upper body backwards whilst exhaling again through the mouth. *Repeat 5–10 times, building up to 50 for strength and endurance work.*

Finish with an All-over stretch.

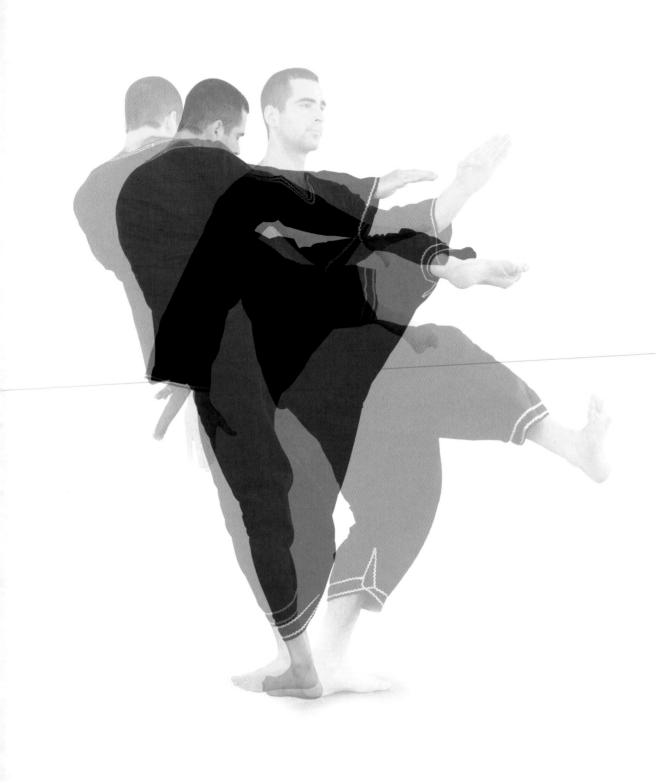

'He was nine years old and finally ready to train with his aunt in the art he was so keen to discover. The boy from Sumatra, Indonesia had learned to imitate the movements of Silat by watching his seniors in the early morning practice. His new teacher had a serene walk as she gracefully approached a small palm. There was silence. Her posture was flawless as her movement exploded like a whirlpool, with perfect co-ordination. He saw, as the tree fell, how she carried her razor sharp Kris dagger – one in each hand...and one in each foot.'

Pentjak Silat, or the Art of Self-defence, has evolved into various styles. Those who live in rocky grounds use an upright stance, whilst those who dwell in the muddy, more

THE CORE >>

slippery landscape crouch low, like a tiger. The fundamentals, however, remain constant. Training begins with ground forms which familiarise the beginner with his 'best-friend' in a combat situation. The forms include a variety of kicks, rolls, evasions and take-downs, and even when the practitioner progresses to a standing stance his power emanates from the ground.

Soft, dance-like forms help to develop the unique Silat 'flow', and jurus, short forms comprising a single attack of four or five strikes, develop speed and power. In order to increase sensitivity, buahs, or partner drills, are practised, with an unremitting emphasis placed on artistic movement as well as effective application. The art of Silat will help us to build a cornerstone of muscle strength, or core stability.

Core stability

After years of doing exercise classes and workout routines in which the emphasis has been on acquiring high levels of aerobic fitness through large dynamic movements, the fitness industry and related research units now recognise and promote the benefits of what is called 'core stability', using small controlled movements to stabilise the torso. The importance of core training has long been understood by dancers, and practitioners of martial arts, yoga and pilates, and its value is now acknowledged as an essential and fundamental part of our physical activity.

Some researchers have described the body's trunk as having an 'inner' unit surrounded by an 'outer' unit. The inner unit includes the transverse abdominals, the diaphragm and the muscles of the pelvic floor. Effective functioning of this unit is considered essential in preventing back

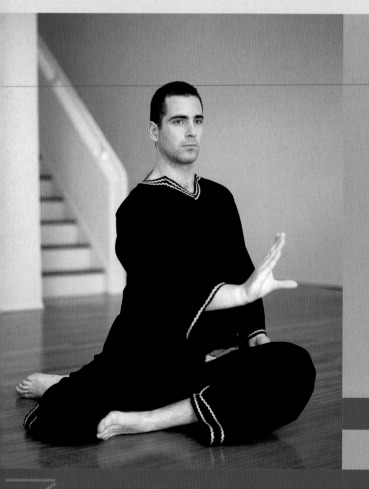

<< THE CORE WORKOUT

If you have always dreamed of a flat stomach, it is not beyond your grasp. The good news is that you don't have to do abdominal workouts daily to see results. Nor do you need to perform countless repetitions either. The exercises in this chapter will strengthen and tone your abdominals and improve your core stability just by doing them two to three times a week.

However doing these exercises alone won't give you a flat stomach. The quality of your diet and the amount of fat-burning aerobic exercise you do is crucial. We all have a 'six-pack' already, but most of them are covered by a layer of fat. So use these exercises as a balanced part of your workout, and you will get the abdominals that you have dreamed of.

EASY ★   MEDIUM ★★   HARD ★★

injury and ensuring optimum performance in activity. The 'outer' unit includes the other abdominal muscles as well as the muscles of the back, pelvis and hip which, working together, contribute to the stabilisation of the pelvic girdle and spine.

So what does this all mean for you and me? It means that however much we might enjoy the high intensity running and jumping around aspects of exercise, there comes a time when we need to get floor-based and spend time working on this 'core stability'. These muscles are some of the hardest working muscles in our bodies. They are our primary source for balance, posture and overall body strength; they deserve our time and attention. In addition, good core stability can mean great-looking abdominals, and who doesn't want that?

Cobra stretch ★

1. Lying on the floor on your stomach, place your hands flat on the floor with your thumbs level with your armpits. Breathing out, raise your head up slowly, arching your back. Try to keep your lower body motionless, heavy and strong. Feel the chest opening and the spine lengthening. Keep the movement slow and sinuous. Hold for 10 seconds and return to the floor.

>>

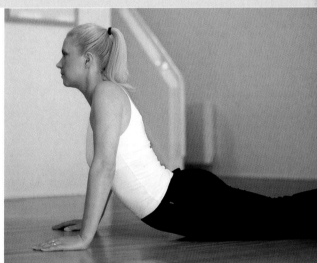

<<

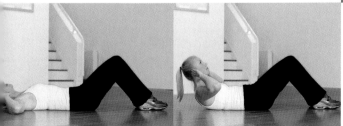

Basic sit-ups ★

1. Lie on your back with your knees bent, and your lower back gently pressed down towards the floor, if necessary, letting your spine find a neutral position. Let your pelvis rise naturally up and tighten your abdominal muscles.

2. Cupping your ears with your hands, and keeping your chin off your chest, breathe out and lift up. Return to the floor slowly and repeat immediately.
Do 15 repetitions and then rest.

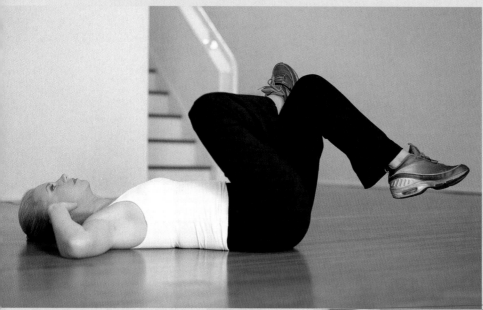

Alternate leg crunch ★★

1. Lie on the floor on your back, and press your lower back into the floor if necessary, making sure your spine is in a neutral position. Place both hands by your ears. Put your right leg over your left (ankle on upper knee) and lift up.

2. Keeping your legs as still as possible, take your left shoulder towards the right knee. Keep your chin off your chest and breathe out as you lift up. To make this easier leave your foot on the floor.

Do 10–15 repetitions on each side.

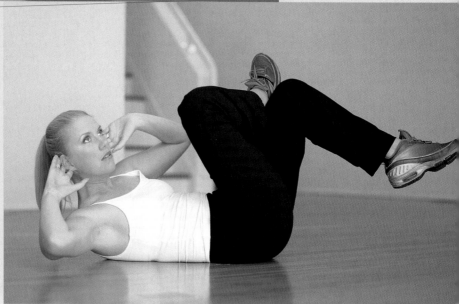

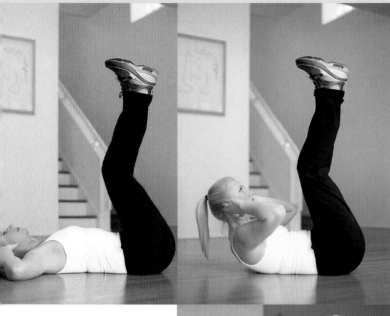

<<

Vertical leg crunch ★★

1. Lie on the floor on your back and raise your legs up, with your lower back gently pressed to the ground and your spine in a neutral position. Knees should be flexed. Cup your ears with your hands and keep your chin off your chest.

2. Breathing out, use your abdominal muscles to lift your head and shoulders. Keep your legs still. Return slowly to the floor and repeat. *Do 15–30 repetitions and then rest.*

Side curls ★★ >>

1. From the above position, raise your legs straight up and cross your ankles. 'Anchor' your lower back into the floor and place your hands by your ears.

2. Breathing out, lift and twist gently taking the right shoulder towards the left knee. Hold this move for 1–2 seconds at the top of the move then return to the floor and repeat the other way. *Do 15–30 repetitions and then rest.*

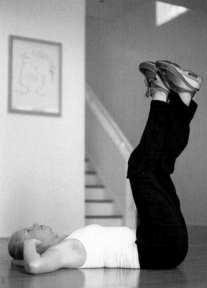
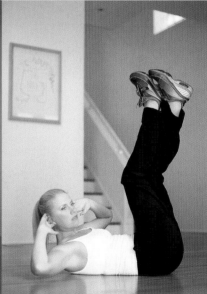

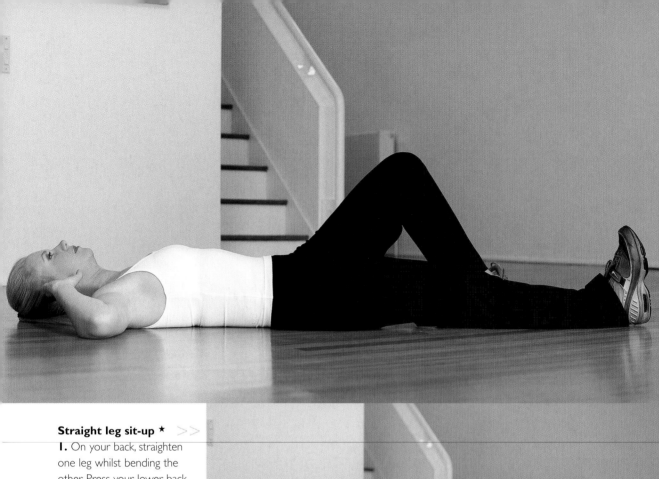

Straight leg sit-up ★ >>

1. On your back, straighten one leg whilst bending the other. Press your lower back gently into the floor, keeping your spine in a neutral position.

2. Cup your ears with your hands, keeping the chin off the chest, and lift up slowly whilst breathing out.

Do 10–15 repetitions with one leg straight, change legs and repeat the same amount of repetitions on the other side immediately.

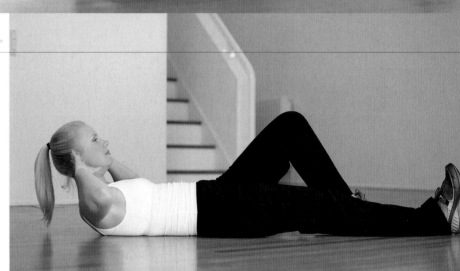

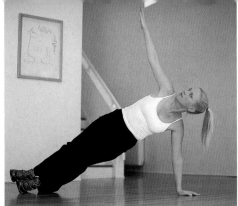

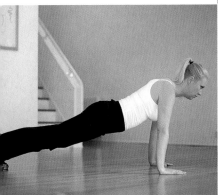

Plank pose moving into side plank★★★

1. Begin on your hands and knees, hands under your shoulders, knees under hips. Walk back until your legs are straight and you are balancing on your toes, feet together. Keep shoulders back and down and arms straight. Do not lock your elbows. Hold for 5 breaths.

2. Squeeze your ankles together, roll to outer edge of the foot, keeping the legs stacked and straight. Lift your right hand towards ceiling; then look towards it. Let your abdominals support your body without clamping. Lower your hand towards the floor, returning to the plank pose.

Repeat on other side. Hold each pose for 5 breath cycles.

Bicycle ★★ >>

1. Lie on the floor with your lower back pressed gently down, then raise your knees and put your feet into the air. Rotate your legs as though you were cycling. Make sure you do not twist or raise your back and keep your abdominals tight at all times.

Spend 30 seconds to start with and slowly build up to 1 minute.

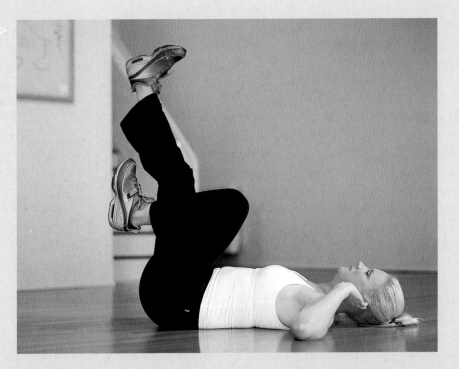

Sit up and hook★★

1. Start on your back with your knees bent and your feet flat on the floor. Gently press your lower back into a neutral spine position. Making soft fists, bend the elbows bringing the arms up towards the chest.

2. Lift through the shoulders and head, squeezing the abdominals, and come up as high as feels comfortable. As you reach the top of the movement throw a right hook immediately followed by a left one. Keep the pace slow to medium, breathing out as you punch. Make sure the work comes from the

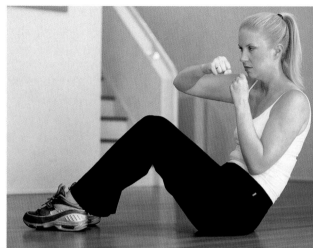

waist, whilst the pelvis remains steadfastly on the floor. Return to the ground and repeat, this time throwing a left hook followed by a right, and so on.
Do a set of 20 repetitions.

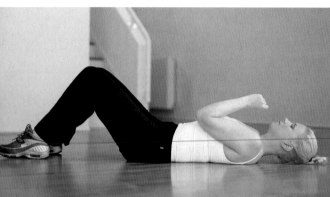

SUGGESTED COMBINATIONS

Easy workout

Basic sit-ups 2 x 15

Cobra stretch

Alternate leg crunch
1 x 15 each way

Intermediate

Vertical leg crunch 2 x 15
working up to 2 x 30

Cobra stretch

Side curls
2 x 15 working up to 2 x 30

Cobra stretch

Straight leg
2 x 20 working up to 2 x 40

Hard

Add to intermediate workout:

Sit up and hook 1 x 20

Plank – side plank 1 x each way

Cobra stretch

Bicycle
2 x 30 seconds working up to
2 x 1 minute

Silat workout

It is virtually impossible to teach Silat conditioning exercises entirely accurately without supervision, however since our aim here is not to master Silat but to help increase our core stability these exercises are highly appropriate and effective.

The Twister   >>

1. Sit with your knees bent and back straight. Now lifting your feet directly off the ground and keeping your knees slightly bent, find your balance point on your lower sacrum. Keeping your abdominal muscles tight, begin to twist from side to side. Concentrate on working through the waist and on keeping your balance. Breathe out as you twist.
Begin with 10 twists and work up to 50.

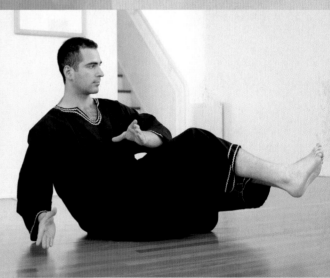

<<

Circles

1. Sit with bent knees and feet on the ground. Tighten through your abdominal muscles and lift your feet off the ground. Find your balance point on your lower sacrum area. Keeping the legs quite relaxed, begin to throw slow perfect circles with alternate legs, with your left leg moving in a clockwise direction and your right leg anti-clockwise. Keep the knees gently flexed and your abdominals tight to help support the back.
Start by doing 10 circles and then work up to 50.

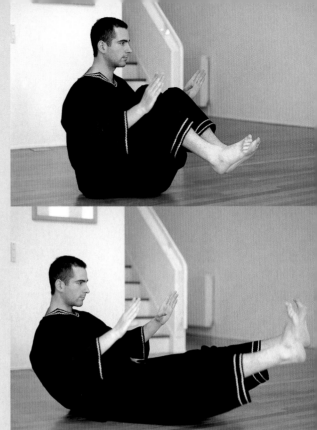

Balanced extensions

1. Sit with your knees bent and your feet flat on the floor. Tighten your abdominals and lift your feet off the floor, balancing on your lower sacrum area. Flex the feet and draw the knees in towards the chest, keeping the abdominals tight to help support the back.

2. Extend both feet, maintaining your balance. Take your legs out until they are straight but not locked at the knee joints. Draw them back in as far as possible and repeat. Exhale as you extend the legs and inhale as you draw them back.

To make this exercise easier, begin by placing your hands parallel to your buttocks, to give you support.

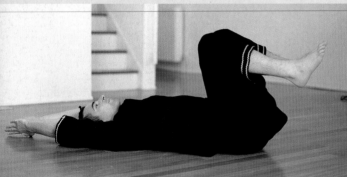

Reverse curl

1. Lie on your back with your knees bent and your feet flat on the floor. Place your hands above your head, with the palms together letting the elbows drop out and relax towards the floor. Lift your feet off the floor bending your knees to approximately 90 degrees. Rest on your tailbone to protect your spine which should be in a neutral position.

2. Using your abdominals, draw the knees up and in, lifting the buttocks off the floor. Take your time – breathe in for a count of 5 on the way up, and 5 on the way down.

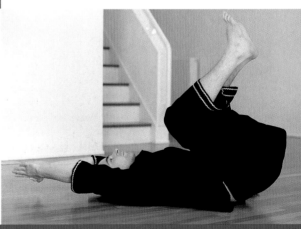

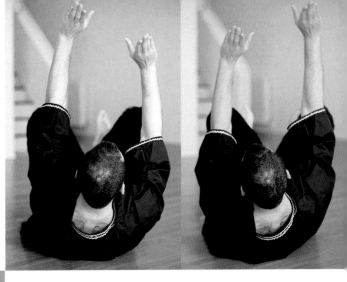

Alternate twist >>

1. Lie on your back with your knees bent and your feet flat on the floor. Lift your feet up off the floor until they are at a 90-degree angle. Make sure your tailbone is in a neutral spine position. Stretch your arms straight up with the palms reaching for the ceiling (and fingers 'pulling' back towards the floor).

2. Inhale, then as you exhale reach further towards the ceiling with alternating palms, twisting through your trunk. Make sure your arms remain straight throughout. Repeat immediately, but still keep it slow, without a breath in between reps.

Perform 3–5 'reaches' on each side all with 1 exhalation and return to ground whilst inhaling.

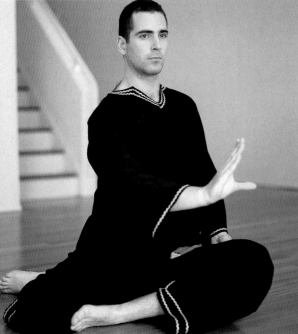

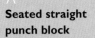

Seated straight punch block

1. Sit as shown with your trunk rotated so that the shoulder of the side of your front leg is rotated backwards.

2. Bend from the waist towards the side of the front leg. As your shoulder approaches your knee twist the body in the opposite direction, towards the ceiling. *Do 20–30 slow repetitions and repeat on the opposite side.*

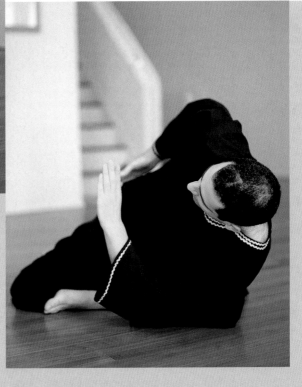

LOWER-BACK WORKOUT

Back extensions

1. Lie on your front and with your arms out sphinx-like to your sides.

2. Keeping your bottom and thighs relaxed, and nose and chest pointing down towards the ground at all times, lift up pushing gently through your forearms. Return to the ground slowly and repeat.

3. To make this harder, place your hands in the small of your back and lift up. Again keep your nose and chest facing down to the ground. This (as the easier version) is quite a small move and is purely trying to target the lower back muscles.

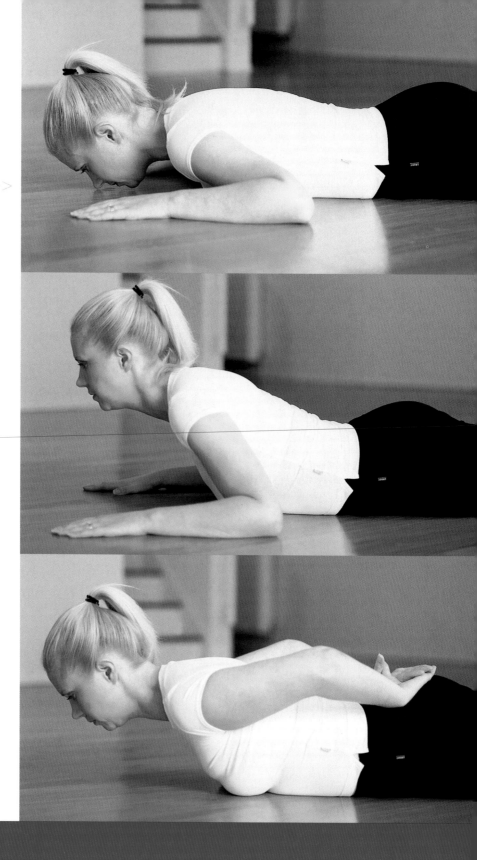

Ball

1. Lie on your back and gently hug your knees into your chest. Make sure your head stays relaxed on the ground. Hold it in this initial position for 10–20 seconds and then begin to rock gently from side to side for another 20 seconds. Don't forget to breathe.

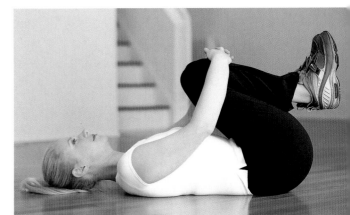

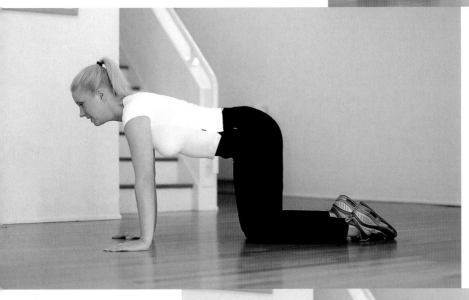

Superman

1. Start on all fours with your hands directly underneath the line of your shoulders and your knees in line with your hips. Tighten your abdominals and keep your back as straight as possible.

2. Lift your right arm and your left leg up in a straight line, then return to the start position and repeat with the left arm and right leg.
Start with 10 repetitions and build up to 20.

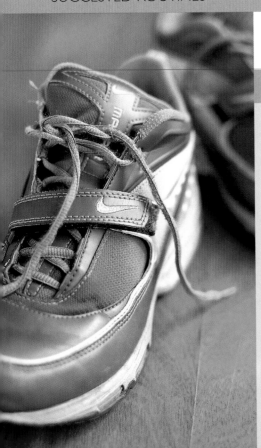

SUGGESTED ROUTINES

Always start off with the 'Easy' routine for the first few sessions.

Easy routine	Medium–hard
Back extension 1 x 15	Back extension 1 x 15–20
Ball	Ball
Back extension 1 x 15	Back extension 1 x 15–20
Ball	Ball
Superman 1 x 10	Superman 1 x 20
	Cat stretch
	Pelvic thrust 1 x 10
	Try finishing any of these workouts with our 'Back and Abdominal stretch'

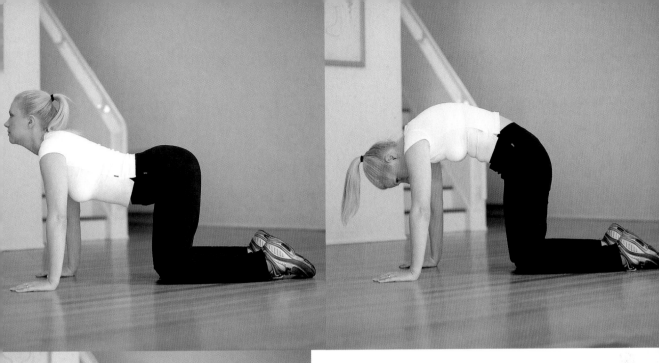

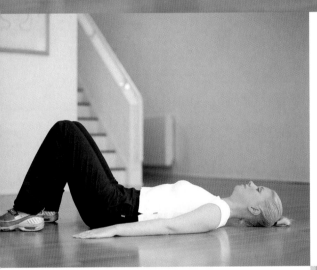

Cat stretch

1. Kneeling on all fours with your hands directly underneath your shoulders and your knees in line with your hips. Relax your fingers by wiggling them and then splaying them out. Begin by curving your back down to hollow it, at the same time lifting your head up.

2. Now arch your back up to hunch it whilst dropping your head. Breathe continuously throughout. *Repeat 10 times.*

Pelvic thrust

1. Lie on your back with your knees bent and your feet hip-width apart.

2. Keeping your feet and shoulders still, raise your pelvis into the air as high as it will go, then lower it one vertebra at a time, beginning at the top and slowly working your way down. *Repeat 10 times.*

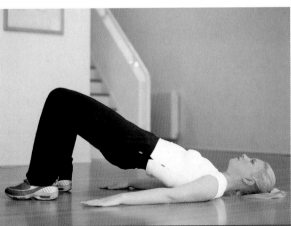

Fight that fat!

You have now got the great abs, but are they still covered in that layer of body fat? More than likely, unfortunately. Body fat has a nasty habit of sticking to where we least want it, and to some degree this is completely beyond our control. Your size and shape are largely down to genetics. By sheer tenacity and with a lot of hard work you can fight against this, but it is extremely hard, not to mention unwise, in the long term and your body will tend to revert back quickly to your inherited shape. Your pre-determined package is usually what you should accept and then do your best with.

The best thing everyone can do for their self-esteem and to build faith in their own body is to throw away the scales. Too many people have become not only a slave to their scales but also addicted to weight/height charts. Neither is an accurate gauge of either fitness or body composition – two women of identical height and weight can look completely different if one is toned and slim, and the other fat and flabby.

The reason for this is that muscle weighs up to three times as much as fat. Many people get disheartened when they start exercising and find they put weight on rather than lose it, but in fact they are getting fitter. As we exercise, our body-fat percentage gets lower and lean muscle is gained, giving us a sleek toned look rather than a wobble. And as lean muscle weighs more than fat, scales (and weight/height charts) fail to give us an accurate picture of the state of our bodies.

So what is body fat?

Body fat is the tissue in and around our muscles that is made up of fat cells, which burns slowly to sustain the body when food is scarce. In the Western world, however, food is rarely scarce, so many of us have too much body fat. These fat cells are used to store energy and cushion the body but, depending on age and gender, it should be no more than 20–30 per cent of the body's composition.

Once you have thrown out your scales, you will need to find another way of monitoring your body fat. One way is to use a favourite piece of clothing. Pick something from a point in your life when you looked and felt great – and you weren't starving yourself or over-exercising. Wear it or try it on every couple of weeks and see how it feels.

Another method is to calculate your body mass index (BMI). However this too can be far from perfect: an extremely muscular person – an elite athlete for example – may have an abnormally high BMI. But it is easy to use and a reasonable indicator of whether you have a weight problem. The official BMI formula is weight in kilograms divided by height in metres squared and the classifications are as indicated in the box above right.

Whilst some experts disagree on where a normal BMI should end and an overweight one should begin, most agree that you should be concerned if your BMI approaches 27. This is because people who are overweight or obese are more likely to develop obesity-related diseases, such as heart disease, diabetes, high blood pressure and some forms of cancer.

There are a number of machines on the market now that have been designed to calculate body fat. These often give a more accurate reading although it varies between make and model. Most health clubs and gyms also offer a body-fat measuring and maintenance service.

Body Mass Index	
Below 18.5	Underweight
18.5–24.9	Normal
25–29.9	Overweight
Over 30	Obese

It is all well and good knowing your body fat percentage, but what can you do to reduce it? Well, don't be tempted to crash diet. The human body does not like to be deprived of food; it goes into starvation mode. Then, as soon as any food is eaten, the body stores it as fat. The key is to eat sensibly and exercise. Toning workouts give you sleek toned muscles. Fat-burning cardiovascular workouts serve to improve your heart and lung capabilities and burn calories. Do a combination of both and over a sensible period of time, watch that excess body fat melt away.

A huge variety of fitness activities provide cardiovascular and fat-burning benefits. If you are breathing hard and you can feel your heart beating you are doing a cardio workout. For the benefit of the workouts in this book I would suggest using one of the following ways to help incorporate a different aerobic technique into your weekly exercise programme.

A long continuous walk

There are many ways to walk. We cannot expect our usual gentle stroll to the shops is going to make a marked difference. We need to challenge the body. Different speeds of walking burn different levels of calories. Even though it may take longer, 1 mile of walking burns the same as 1 mile of jogging. Walking a gentle 3mph burns 70 calories in 2 minutes. But doing 4.5mph for 20 minutes burns 90 calories, a 20 per cent increase. So keep that walking brisk.

As with anything that you begin, start off slowly. Begin with 10 minutes of easy walking to warm up. Take it at a pace that's slow enough to be comfortable but will also gently increase your level of breathing. Cool down in the same fashion. This walking workout should be challenging yet comfortable. The idea is to get your heart pumping and yourself sweating. However you should not let yourself get out of breath. The guideline is that you should be able to maintain a conversation – this is called a 'talk test'. If you find yourself getting out of breath, slow down the pace a fraction and let yourself recover.

When your fitness levels have improved by walking on the flat, the next step is to add some hills. Even a modestly steep incline can increase calorie burn by 30 per cent. Find yourself a hill. Climb at a hard pace for 2 minutes, then turn back round and walk back down the hill at an easy pace. Repeat this cycle 6 to 8 times.

Correct posture list

Head and neck. Keep your head centred between your shoulders, with your neck relaxed Shoulders and chest. Your shoulders should be down and relaxed. Chest and ribcage should be 'lifted'.

Arms and hands. Bend your elbows to 90 degrees. Cup your hands gently keeping them relaxed. Drive your elbows back as you walk, letting them skim the body; to go faster, pump your arms a bit quicker and your legs will follow.

Abs and lower back. Pull your abdominal muscles in but don't hold your breath!

Legs and feet. Power leg movements from the hips. Keep your knees soft. Relax your ankles. Put your heel down first and roll through – heel, ball and toe.

When you have mastered walking, you could now begin to add small jogs into your workout. If you have never run or jogged before, begin slowly. Try doing your normal warm-up and then add one minute of slow jogging into your walk. For example: do a ten-minute warm-up walk, jog for one minute, walk for two to three minutes, jog for one minute and so on. As you get used to jogging you can increase the running time as you wish until you get to a point where you don't need to walk at all. However do make sure you begin and end your jog and/or run with a walking section.

VARIED PACE RUNNING

Our final idea combines aerobic work such as running with faster running or short sprints. Working aerobically (with oxygen) and anaerobically (without oxygen) helps to improve the speed of recovery and the body's ability to maximise oxygen intake. The long and short of it is, it will improve your stamina and burn calories. An established form of this varied pace running is called fartlek, a Swedish word meaning 'speed-play'. As with everything we have done, take everything at your own pace – don't run before you can walk.

Try this typical fartlek session:

1. Jogging (5 minutes)
2. A fast, evenly paced run (3 minutes)
3. Brisk walk (2 minutes)
4. Evenly paced running with 50–60 metre sprints every 200 metres (5 minutes)
5. Jogging (5 minutes)
6. Evenly paced running with occasional inclusion of 4–5 fast strides – small accelerated sprints (3 minutes)
7. Jogging with one fast uphill run – 20–30 metres – every minute (5 minutes)
8. Jogging and rhythmical exercises, skipping and knee raises (5 minutes)

Cool down with a brisk walk and don't forget to stretch!

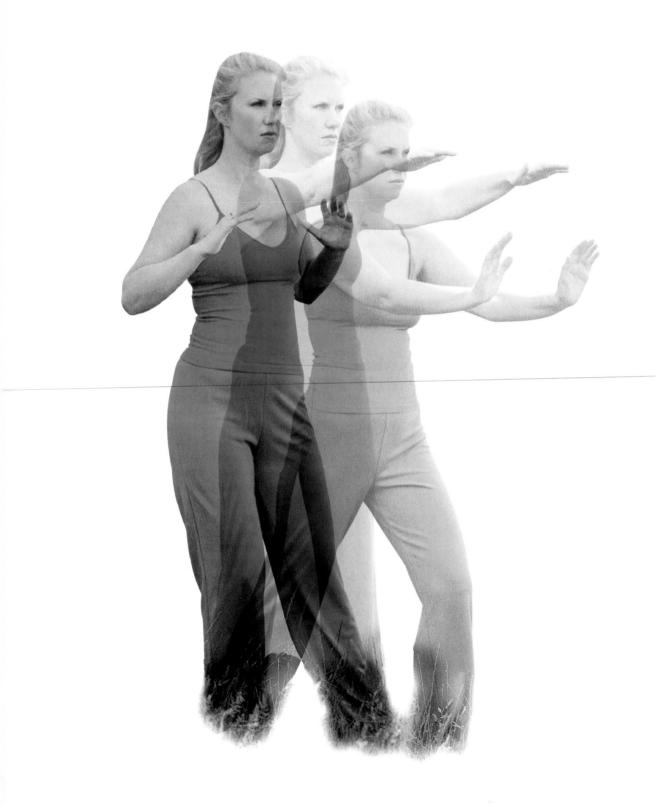

Tai chi is a system of exercises and movements to promote health and longevity, and though it might not look like it at first glance, it is a comprehensive system of self-defence. Its roots are in China, where it evolved over many hundred years as a martial art, and as a system of self-development.

It has become a multi-dimensional art form that has the capacity to touch on several levels the life of anybody who embarks on its exploration. Tai chi is not just about health or about self-defence, but about the development of the whole individual – body, mind and spirit.

THE DE-STRESS ZONE >>

Tai chi shapes and reshapes the body's energy field, keeping its channels clear and energising them. It opens up exciting possibilities for change to be brought about consciously through working with different aspects of the body. However it is not essential to know a great deal about meridians or energy centres in order to practise tai chi. By practising on a regular basis you should start to feel and witness the changes it can bring within your own energy patterns and emotional well-being.

The aim of the workouts in the De-Stress Zone is to give you a wide variety of reasons and choices to slow down, relax and de-stress using a combination of tai chi, chi kung and various meditation techniques.

Getting started

These exercises are designed to increase body awareness and relaxation. Try them whenever you have ten minutes to spare and you are feeling the need to relax, take stock and de-stress.

Standing like a mountain between heaven and earth

This exercise aims to raise your awareness of the relationship between the parts of the body and their alignment from the feet on the earth to the head in the sky. Through this the hip joints are being asked to 'soften' and to open up whilst gently stretching. Your knees should be sensitive to their own alignment, since they act as channels allowing the force of gravity to pass through. The positioning of the feet affects the whole alignment of the frame, from which descends an imaginary channel that anchors the body to the earth's centre.

1 Firstly stand comfortably with your feet well apart. Start to notice how and where the weight of your body comes down through your feet. Is it towards your toes or the heels, the instep of the outside of your foot, or just somewhere in the middle?

2 Now begin to rock your weight slowly forwards to the front of your feet and then back. Repeat 2–3 times. When you stop, allow the feet to meet the earth fully, with your weight now evenly balanced.

3 Bring your weight to the instep. You should immediately feel an unwanted strain on your knees. This is because they are now misaligned and not designed to work properly in this position. Redistribute your weight evenly across your feet.

4 Realign your knees so they follow the direction of your feet. This maintains the correct relationship between the feet, the knees and the heels. Try to feel it by dropping your spine a few inches. Look down to make sure your kneecap follows in line with your toes.

5 Stand upright again. Turn your feet to point slightly outwards and then once again drop your spine and bend your knees. Check that your knees are in line with your toes. Notice the effect on your hips whilst you are doing this.

6 Keeping your legs and upper body still, rock your pelvis backwards and forwards, then from side to side. Try to imagine your pelvis 'floating'. Circle it a few times in each

direction. Feel the link between your lower pelvis and your hip joints, and the relationship between your pelvis and your feet.

7 Drop the spine and softly bending the knees, open and soften the hips. Repeat this move a few times allowing the hips to move and open. Feel the connection between your feet, knees and hips. Your feet should be anchored to give you stability, your hips to allow mobility.

8 With your feet planted on the ground and your weight distributed evenly so that your knees and toes are aligned, and your pelvis free to move, feel as though your spine is carrying your neck up towards the sky. Now try to drop

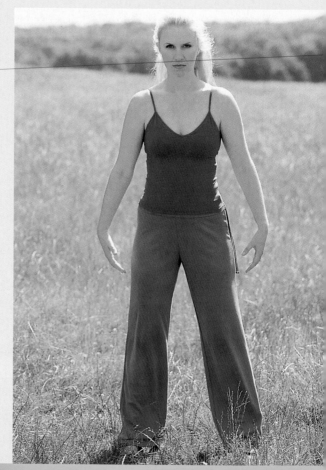

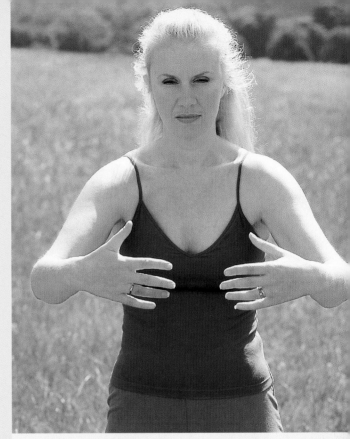

your spine to sit into the earth, relaxing your muscles downward (yin) whilst simultaneously feel the upward and outward support of your bones (yang).

9 Lift your arms out a little way from your body. Imagine your shoulder joints opening, letting in space. As you do this, feel your arms lift further out. Begin to explore all the movement possibilities of your elbows, then your wrists, then turn your fingertips up towards each other. Imagine your arms are growing out from your spine, and make a connection with your fingers.

10 Finally direct your attention to the top of your head. Soften the muscles here and downwards through your whole body. At the same time imagine the bones of your spine lifting you to this point. Feel the polarity between your feet in the earth and your head in the sky. This should keep your spine open and stretched up and down, so that it falls into its natural curved shape.

Holding a ball

From the above position go into the position of Holding a ball, in which you should relax and hold up to any comfortable length of time. Since a beginner to this position finds it hard to learn to relax, you might only be able to hold this position comfortably for 20–30 seconds to start with. However as you begin to let go physically and mentally, you will find that the time that you can stand in this position increases dramatically.

1. Stand with your feet apart, toes pointing forwards and slightly inwards, and the knees slightly bent. Keep your upper body straight. Raise the arms to shoulder level with the palms facing you, fingers slightly apart. Bend and drop the elbows slightly as if you were holding a large beach ball against your chest. Breathe deeply, closing the eyes if you wish.

2. Alternatively, move the arms as if you were holding the ball with one arm on top and one arm below.

>>

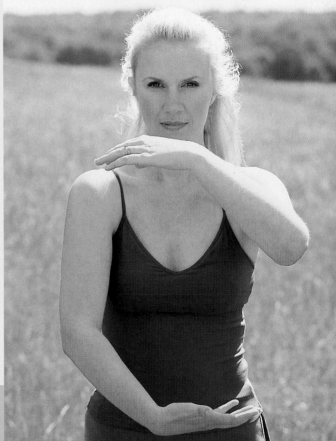

The de-stress workout

PREPARATION FOR PRACTICE

When working through any tai chi or chi kung sequence your attention needs to be in many places at once. Before you begin, spend a few minutes attuning yourself physically and mentally to what you are about to do. Stand and work through these points:

>> The higher extension point lies roughly 18 inches above the head, bordering the aura that surrounds the body. It links the cosmos to the body and indirectly the earth through the spine and pelvis. Start by directing your awareness to this point, as you do so you should 'feel' your spirit lifting through the top of your head.

>> The top of the head is linked by the spine to the coccyx joining the spirit of the universe to the matter of the earth. Feel it as soft and lifted from above. Directing your awareness to this helps to maintain a dynamic and live pathway along the spine.

>> The sacrum is the lower part of the spine that is built into the pelvis. In tai chi it connects the spine to the earth, symbolised by the legs and feet. Directing your awareness to the sacrum makes for effective grounding.

>> The hands are your sensors in tai chi – they are your antennae. Always be aware of this primary function, as givers and receivers.

>> The lower tantien energy centre lies halfway between the top of the head and the feet. Focusing attention here awakens its role as the distributor of chi.

>> The feet are terminals through which the body becomes a conductor for power from the Earth. Imagine a gateway through each foot. Directing the attention to the legs and feet encourages earthing.

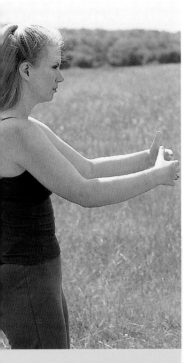

<<

Sunrise
A morning revitalise workout to lighten and refresh your spirit for the day ahead – try doing this workout before breakfast.

Stand with your weight distributed evenly and your feet shoulder-width apart. Spend a few minutes in preparation practice.

1. Sit deeply into both of your feet and slowly raise your hands to chest level, imagining that you are lifting the sun from under the earth up through your feet.
2. Imagine the sun filling your heart and that its light floods through your whole body and bursts out to shine in the space around you. Raise your hands and face towards the sky.
3. Relax your face and turn forwards, and, lowering your arms, open them fully so they extend upwards and outwards. Stand and enjoy this position of radiance. Finish by centring yet again.
Repeat steps 1–3 twice more.

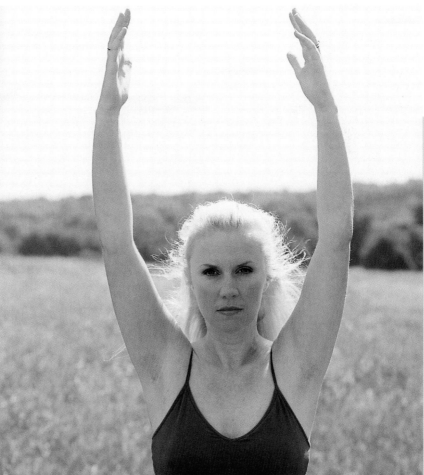

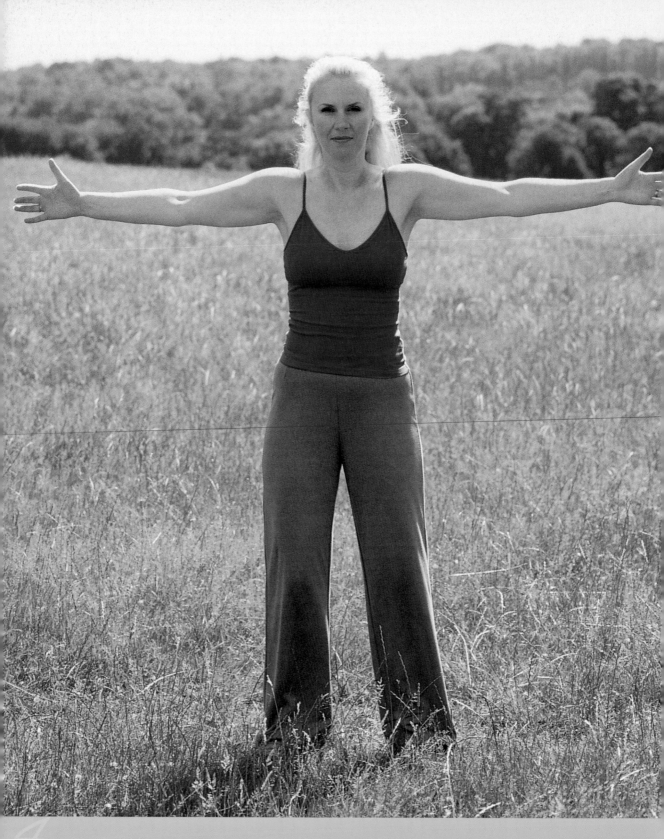

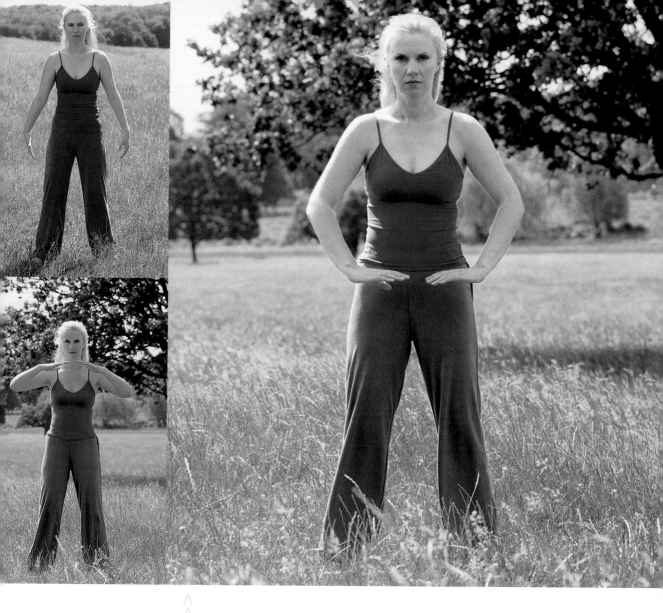

Sunset

An evening de-stress workout to leave you feeling quiet, contained and peaceful at the end of the day. You could either try this when you get in from work to help you unwind or use it just before you go to bed.

1. Begin by standing with your weight distributed evenly and your feet shoulder-width apart. Spend a few minutes going through your preparation for practice sequence.

2. Circle your arms upwards in a large arc, finishing with your fingertips about 2 inches (5cm) apart by your face.

Feel a sense of 'gathering'.

3. Move your hands slowly and gracefully down to rest by your sides like the sun setting.

Repeat the 3 steps twice more. Now rest your hands on your lower dan tian, imagining all your energy centres alive and balanced.

Short chi kung – dao yin workout

Try to practise the following exercises for a few minutes every day, concentrating only on your moves, your inner calmness, and banish all other worries and fleeting thoughts.

Adjusting the breath
1. Stand with your feet shoulder-width apart, toes pointing forwards and slightly inwards. Keep the body straight and the pelvis tucked under. Your hands are at your side and the shoulders slightly rounded.
2. Slowly lift up your arms (imagine you are moving through water) keeping the move fluid and soft. Take the arms to just below shoulder height and return slowly down. Repeat this move 8 times. Breathe in and out through the nose. Each arm lift should take 5–6 seconds.

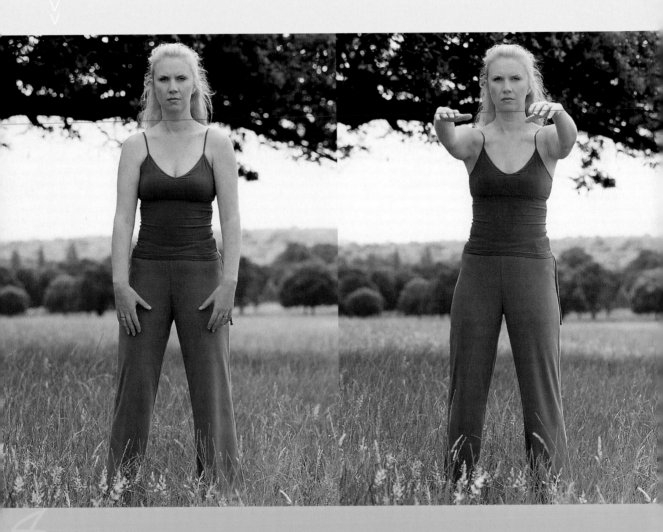

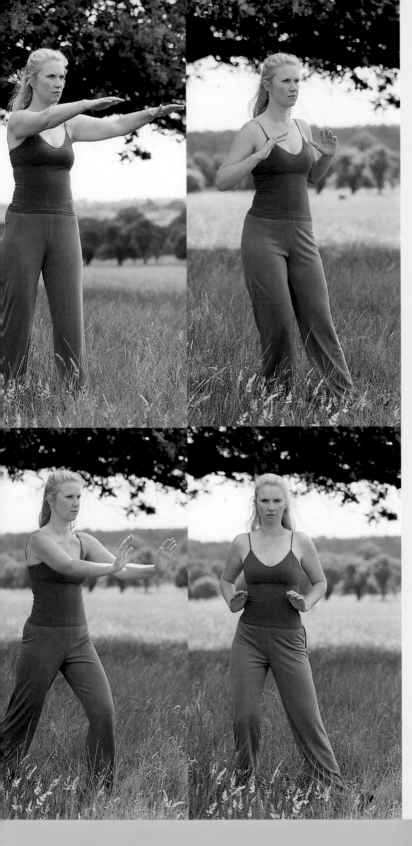

<<

Pushing the boat out

1. Keeping the legs and hips in the same position, turn the waist to the left whilst lifting the arms.

2. Now turn the hips back to the centre drawing in the elbows whilst dropping the hands. Sink body weight on to right foot.

3. Turn the hips and body to the left 45 degrees and then pick up the left leg placing the heel on the floor. Push forwards with the heel of the palms and sink 70 per cent of your body weight on to the front foot.

4. Turn hips and body to the front sinking weight into right foot. Arms come round and are drawn into the body whilst lifting left foot off the floor.

Repeat steps 3 and 4 once more. Return to centre and repeat other way.

Shouldering the moon and the sun

1. Start with your feet together. Now slowly rotate to the left lifting your arms with the palms facing up (imagine you are carrying small candles). As you twist your torso, let your head look behind.

2. Turn back to the centre bringing the arms forwards and up (don't let that candle drop!).

3. Press the hands back down to the start position and repeat to the right. *Repeat 4 times in each direction.*

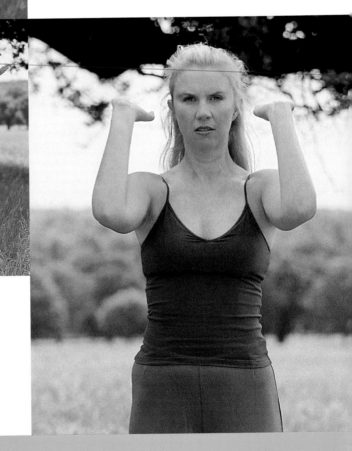

Meditation

Some of the chi kung exercises that we have looked at can be considered a moving meditation. But as with everything de-stressing and meditating is a very personal state, and what works perfectly for one person might not work for the other. Other forms of meditation include seated static ones and there are various methods that you can make your own.

Meditation is an ancient discipline that involves contemplation whilst focusing your mind on a thought or an object. It is a practice that is said to help you understand everything in your life more clearly. Another description would be to call meditation relaxation – a conscious and chosen relaxation that you can dip in and out of when you feel you need to take a personal time-out from the world. Meditative practices are part of many religious and martial art traditions. There are several common principles: outwardly, an awareness of posture, breath, and mental control; inwardly, a spiritual search. If you are not drawn to its religious or spiritual purposes, do remember it can also be used simply as a valuable time to stop, think and examine your world around you. We are all moving too fast too often, and spending time meditating is a wonderful way to get back in touch with your own directions and principles.

So how do I get started?

First you need to create the right environment. Ideally you would pick a quiet place within your home that you can return to regularly. This space should be pleasant, naturally lit, the right temperature and clean. If you have a peaceful garden where you feel totally undisturbed, then this could become an ideal fair-weather place. How you sit is again an individual choice, as long as you are comfortable and not distracted by lumpy carpets or squeaky chairs. Try a hard-backed chair or a comfortable rug or cushion. Finally do your best to avoid distractions; for example, take the phone off the hook. Try not to worry about too much external noise, you will learn to block this out whilst meditating.

Becoming relaxed is the best preparation for meditation. It is very important to be sitting comfortably. If you find yourself in an uncomfortable position, you will be easily distracted and prone to fidgeting. Traditional, cross-legged postures are perfect for long periods of sitting, but can be hard if you are not supple. Try to keep your back straight and your shoulders pulled gently back. You could also try kneeling on a cushion on a low bench. Finally either clasp your hands or place them gently in your lap to stop them fidgeting.

Start breathing slowly and deeply. Try repeating the following words to yourself, and start to feel the tension release: 'The muscles of my neck are relaxing: I am relaxed. The muscles of my shoulders and chest are relaxing: I am relaxed. The muscles of my arms and hands are relaxing: I am relaxed. The muscles of my legs and feet are relaxing: I am relaxed. My mind is calm. My body is calm. I am relaxed. My mind is alert. My mind is awake.'

Now you are relaxed outwardly, you can begin to meditate inwardly. Meditation is inwardly active. Your mind must keep focused on its subject. This means following wanted thoughts while letting unwanted ones pass. Following a thought requires concentration. For example imagine yourself exploring an ancient castle with many rooms and doors. Eventually come to a door with your name

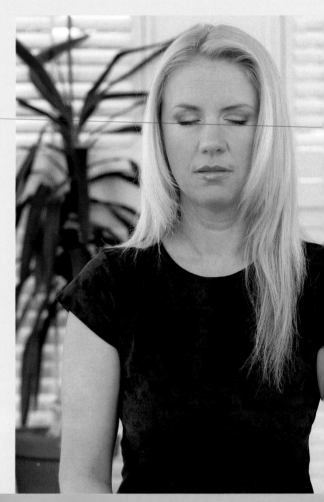

on it. Opening it, you find a spiral staircase. Descend the staircase taking each step slowly. Take your time. Use all your senses to imagine the scene clearly. This staircase can take you deeply into yourself, since it represents the whole you. Reverse your journey to end the meditation.

There are many other things you can visualise, some may be appropriate for you personally. How about a walk in sun-filled woods or a stroll along a lapping shoreline? Choose a place that fills you with harmony and relaxation. Five minutes daily is a good start. Longer sessions will not necessarily provide more benefit than a short one, especially when you have just begun to meditate. However if daily is just not feasible then something is always better than nothing. After a while, you will probably sit for longer periods, and discover a pattern that suits you best.

You can also try this tai chi standing meditation at any point during the day. As with a seated one, find a quiet place where you will be undisturbed. Take the phone off the hook and, if necessary, put a 'do not disturb' sign on the door

1. Stand comfortably with your feet shoulder width apart. Slowly rock back and forth, from the balls to the heels of your feet. Repeat several times, finishing with a more even sense of weight distribution.

2. Bring your awareness to the base of your spine (your sacrum), perhaps resting the back of your hand there. Feel the triangle made by your right foot, your left foot and your sacrum, and imagine it as your base.

3. Imagine gateways into the earth passing through your feet. Through them your consciousness can move into the earth, and the earth into you.

4. Take your awareness from your sacrum down through your right leg and foot to the earth centre. Then raise it again through your left foot back to the sacrum. Repeat four times.

5. Soften the top of your head (think of it relaxing). Feel its link with your sacrum and the connection between your sacrum, feet and earth. Feel a connection from the earth's centre to the top of your head.

6. Imagine your arms are rooted in your spine and that they branch out opening at the shoulder, elbow and wrist joints, and into the hands.

7. Make a space between each finger and relax the soft flesh around the hard bones of your hands feeling the contrast.

8. Point your hands towards the ground and imagine your fingers having roots that extend into the earth.

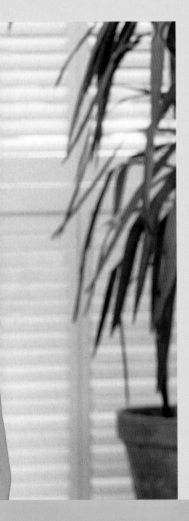

More ideas for mind-body relaxation

DEEP BREATHING

Breathing is the most natural thing in the world. It is instinctive and involuntary and yet how often do you let it work naturally? Most people when asked to breathe a 'full' breath can't – they simply don't know how. Try this simple deep-breathing exercise and feel the difference – place one hand on your upper chest and other on your abdomen for a moment. You will probably just feel a slight rise and fall. Now take a very long deep breath through your nose so you feel your diaphragm descending and your abdomen rising. As you breathe out, the reverse happens.

If you feel meditation isn't for you, then deep-breathing exercises definitely are. They are perfect for relaxation, for centring your thoughts and can be done anywhere.

THE WHISPERED 'AH'

This exercise from the Alexander Technique is a great way of learning to be aware of your breath. It can be done sitting or standing, but is probably better if you stand. As with meditating first find a quiet and warm spot, where you will not be disturbed. To start, mentally scan your body with this checklist in mind:

• Weight should be evenly balanced over your feet, your ankles soft.
• Knees should be relaxed, not locked out.
• Hips should be relaxed, pelvis dropping freely towards floor.
• Abdominal muscles should be relaxed.
• Shoulders should be dropped with the arms hanging free.
• Neck should be relaxed. This can be done by dropping your nose very slightly and imagining someone gently pulling you up from the crown of your head.

Once you have been through the checklist, let your jaw drop open, with your tongue resting lightly behind your lower teeth. Think of something pleasant and smile a little. Now, breathe out gently on a whispered 'Ah', until you have run out of air. There should be very little sound. If you hear any vocalised sound, you are probably holding on to some tension.

Close your mouth. Instead of immediately breathing in, think of doing nothing, and you will notice that your ribs spring out of their own accord. Repeat this process five times. You might find yourself getting a little dizzy. If you do, stop for a moment before continuing.

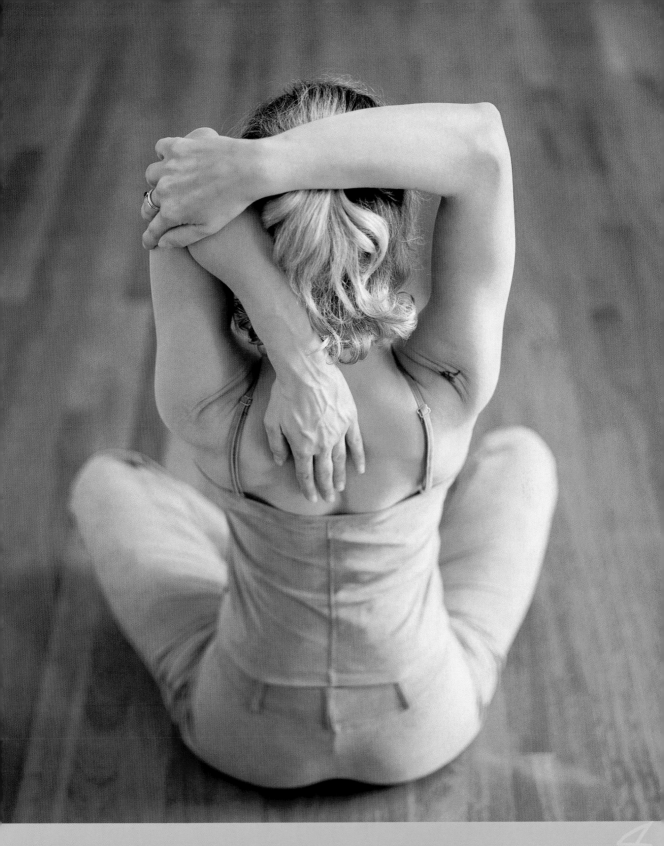

Self-massage

We don't always have either the finances or the person to give us a much needed massage. If you can, treat yourself to a monthly massage, think of it as being part of your whole body care. Not only is it physically good for you, undoing tension points and soothing tired muscles, it is also good for the soul.

However in the interim, try some of these Chinese self-massage treatments. The purpose is to promote harmony of body and mind by stabilising the yin and yang polarity. This is achieved by selecting and massaging acupoints that will regulate the energies of the main meridians. Doing this has a toning, revitalising, strengthening, calming and centring effect on the whole body – what more could you ask for!

>>

Hitting the arms and thighs

1. Sit on a straight-backed chair or on the floor. Using your fist hit along the length of your right arm with the left fist 10 times. Repeat on the other arm. Repeat along the length of the thighs.

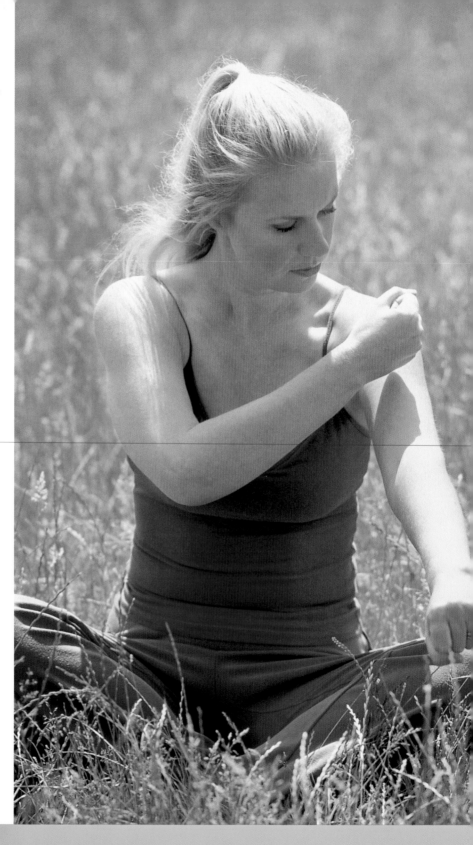

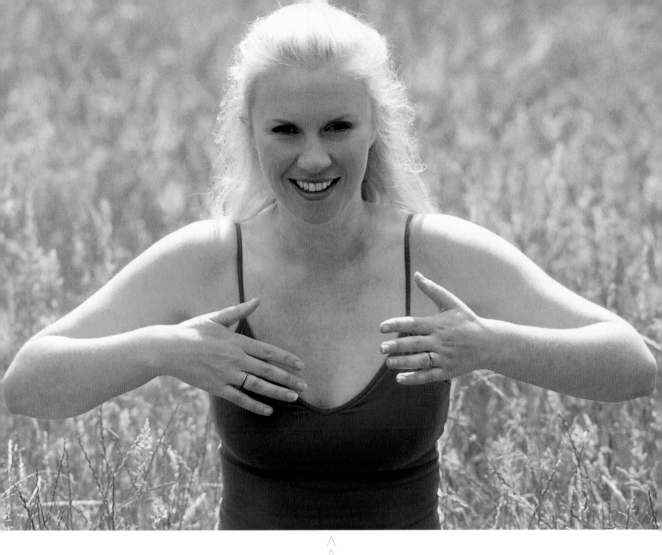

Massaging the shoulders and legs

Still seated, stroke and knead the muscles around the left shoulder joint with the right hand for 1 or 2 minutes. Repeat on the other side. Now rub the surface of the left knee with both hands for 2 minutes, then knead the back of the left knee for 1 minute. Repeat on the other leg. Finally rub the left ankle joint with both hands for 2 minutes. Repeat on the other side.

Patting the chest

Spread the fingers of both hands and tap against the chest with the flats of the fingers, inhaling with each tap. Do this about 7–8 times.

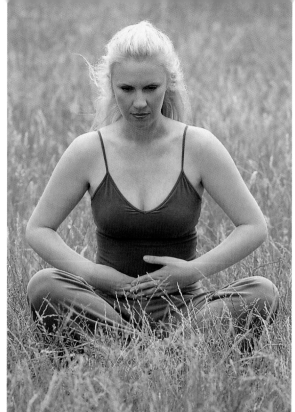

<<

Stroking the dan tian

The dan tian is a traditional acupoint located about 2 inches below the umbilicus. In practice, stroking the dan tian is almost the same as stroking the lower abdomen. Sitting cross-legged, the massage is performed with three fingers of the right hand. Continue for five minutes. This acupuncture point is indicated in cases of indigestion and lower abdominal pain, and has been observed to help relieve such symptoms.

>>

Stroking the kidney point

Rub the hands together to warm the palms. Then stroke the lower back with both hands for five minutes. This point (the shen shu) is located in the lower back. Massaging on this point has a preventative and therapeutic effect for backache.

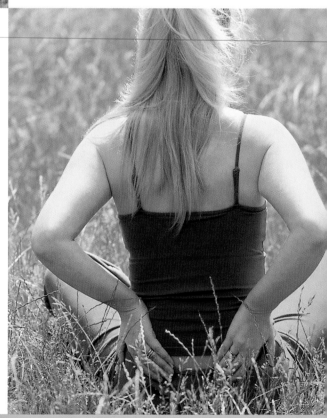

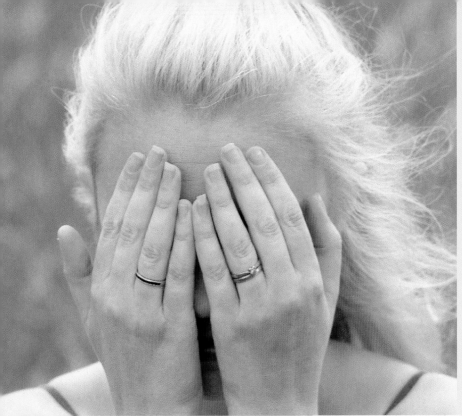

<<

Washing the face

1. Rub your palms together 30–40 times, with increasing speed, until they become warm. Now starting at the base of your chin, run your fingertips and then palms up your face and into your hair line. Do this 5–6 times.

Eye massage

1. Stroke and press the region all around your eyes in a circular motion with the index and middle fingers of both hands.

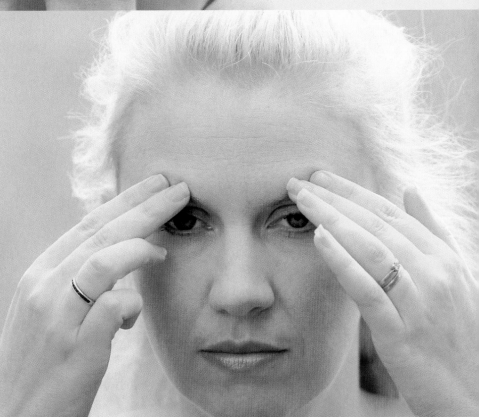

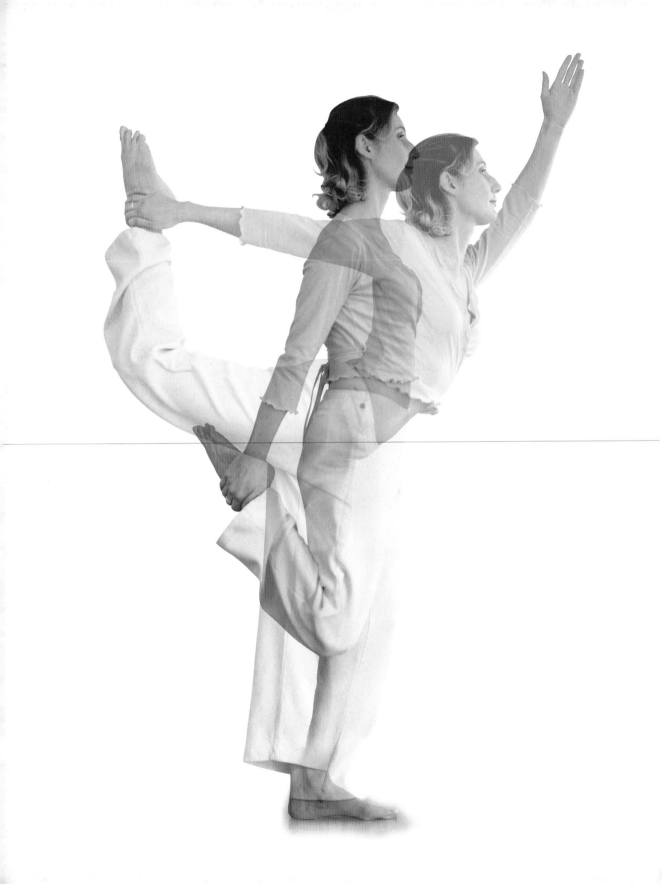

'Prevention is better than cure' is a fundamental precept of all holistic exercise. From the point of view of an exercise teacher or a massage therapist, the majority of injuries can be avoided with a bit of forward planning. Obviously if we are unlucky enough to fall over a broken paving stone or are involved in any form of accident, the related injuries are not self-inflicted.

THE HEALING HAND >>

However back pain, for example, can often be eased by simple stretching and strengthening exercises. Indeed, one of the most consistent factors of all martial arts is the importance of stretching and mobilising muscle groups. Stretching not only improves exercise technique and maintains everyday mobility but it is incredibly important in aiding injury prevention and helping to rebalance the body. It is an essential part of our holistic workout.

Explaining stretching

There are several different types of stretching. The main two are ballistic and static. Ballistic stretching usually involves the performance of bouncing or jerking movements, with the aim being to use the momentum generated to take the body parts involved through a greater range of movement. In general it is not advised since it can increase the risk of injury although it does have its place within certain sports and activities if done correctly and well supervised. For our purposes we will concentrate on static stretching and yoga-based positions.

Static stretching involves moving into the required position at the start of the stretch and holding that position for a set period of time. It can be broken down into maintenance and developmental stretches. Maintenance stretching seeks to maintain your current level of flexibility. This is the type of short stretches (holding in position for roughly 10 seconds) is used after muscle groups have been 'warmed up' to prepare them for the work to come. There has been some research recently arguing against any benefits of a short stretch. However the general consensus is still to include them within all workouts until further research has been concluded. Developmental stretching aims to develop your current level of flexibility. For example, if you are unable to touch your toes at present, a developmental hamstring stretch (rear of thigh muscle) should improve your flexibility and perhaps allow you to do this in future. These stretches take place at the end of our workouts when the body is at its warmest and are held for 20–30 seconds apiece.

BENEFITS OF STRETCHING

>> Improved quality of life. The more flexible you are, the more capable you are of carrying out daily tasks such as bending, stretching and lifting. Reaching down to tie your laces or reaching for tins on the top shelf becomes easier.

>> Improved performance in sport. Flexibility exercises increase the range of movement at a joint, allowing muscles to exert more force over an extended period of time. In golf and tennis for instance, increased flexibility in the shoulder, elbow and waist could enable you to hit the ball harder by generating more force through a greater range of movement.

>> Improved posture. For example, tight hamstrings (rear of thighs) can sometimes pull the pelvis out of alignment and cause an arching of the lower spine. Tight chest muscles can pull the shoulders forwards and cause a rounded upper back.

>> Reduced back pain. Chronic back pain is all too common in the Western world and inflexible hamstrings, hips and lower spine muscles can contribute to this problem. Regular stretching can help to alleviate some problems linked with back pain.

>> Stress management. Stretching can produce profound changes in mental and physical health. Some stress management experts incorporate stretching in their programmes to nurture a calm and relaxed state.

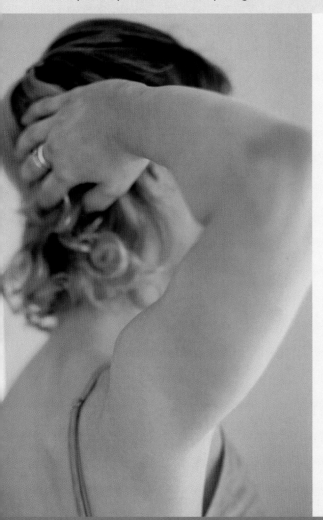

WHEN AND HOW SHOULD I STRETCH?

>> Never compete. We all have different levels of flexibility so always work to your own level.

>> Don't stretch to the point of pain. You should only feel mild discomfort.

>> Always stretch when your muscles are warm. At the end of a workout or after a warm-up are the most suitable times.

>> If you are doing developmental stretches, don't try to do too much too soon. Your body will gradually become more flexible over time, so be patient.

>> Try to get at least three stretching sessions in per week.

>> Aim for balance in your stretches. Don't just do the back of your thighs, for example, balance it out by stretching the front too.

>> Encourage deep, calm and rhythmic breathing.

>> If you are doing a long cool-down stretch, don't get cold. Aim to have clothing to slip on to keep yourself warm throughout.

Many of us have existing injuries and it is a rare person who is 100 per cent fit on starting an exercise programme, so we need to address these problems head-on before we take on a new regime. There are a number of healing arts: here are three of the most interesting and effective complementary methods.

Osteopathy

Osteopathy's origins date back to the nineteenth century with the work of Andrew Taylor Still, a doctor born in 1828 in Virginia, USA. Trained as a doctor according to the system of medical education available at the time, he began to follow a different path from many of his peers. He eschewed alcohol and the habit of contemporary physicians of administering the crude drugs at their disposal in large quantities. Instead he sought new methods of treating sickness. The outcome of his research was the application of physical treatment for which he coined the term 'Osteopathy'.

Now osteopathy is an established and recognised system of diagnosis and treatment, which lays its main emphasis on the structural and functional integrity of the body. It is distinctive in that it recognises that much of the pain and disability that we suffer stems from abnormalities in the function of the body structure as well as damage caused by disease.

Back pain is one of the most common problems for which people seek help from osteopathy, but it can also help with a wide variety of problems including changes to posture in pregnancy, babies with colic or sleeplessness, repetitive strain injury, postural problems caused by driving or work strain, the pain of arthritis and sports injuries among many others.

Your first visit to an osteopath comprises a full case history and an examination. You will normally be asked to remove some of your clothing and to perform a simple series of movements. The osteopath will then use a highly developed sense of touch, called palpation, to identify any points of weakness or excessive strain throughout the body. Further sessions will include the osteopath working with their hands using a wide variety of treatment techniques. These may include soft-tissue techniques, rhythmic passive joint mobilisation or the high velocity thrust techniques designed to improve mobility and the range of movement of a joint. Gentle release techniques are also widely used, especially when treating children or the elderly.

To be sure that you are in safe hands when visiting an osteopath, make sure you use a registered osteopath who will have demonstrated to the General Osteopathic Council via a detailed application process that they are a safe and competent practitioner, that they have adequate insurance and have agreed to abide by a Code of Practice.

Shiatsu

Shiatsu is the traditional hands-on Japanese healing therapy. The philosophy underlying it is that vital energy ('ki' in Japanese) flows throughout the body in a series of channels known as meridians. For many reasons ki can stop flowing freely and this then produces a symptom. A shiatsu practitioner will consider your state of health, the symptoms you are experiencing and, depending on your constitution and general energy levels, will use a wide variety of techniques designed to improve your energy flow. Shiatsu is a deeply relaxing experience and regular sessions are said to help prevent the build-up of stress caused by daily life.

Most sessions last approximately one hour. However the first session might take slightly longer since your chosen practitioner will want to take a detailed case history to help develop a complete picture of your health according to the principles of oriental medicine. The session usually takes place on a padded mat or futon at floor level, although it is possible to receive shiatsu seated if you are unable to lie down. The client stays fully clothed and the practitioner uses a variety of techniques which could include gentle holding, pressing with palms, thumbs, fingers, elbows and knees on the meridians and, when appropriate, more synamic rotations and stretches. Following a treatment, there should be a feeling of increased vitality and you should feel invigorated yet relaxed.

The Shiatsu Society maintains a register of qualified practitioners, each of whom has been assessed for professionalism and clinical expertise by a panel of highly respected practitioners and teachers of shiatsu.

Reiki

Reiki is a Japanese form of healing that is becoming increasingly popular world-wide. In Japanese it means 'spirit-led life-force energy'. What makes reiki unique is that it incorporates elements of just about every other alternative healing practice such as spiritual healing, auras, crystals, chakra balancing, meditation, aromatherapy, naturopathy and homeopathy.

It involves the transfer of energy from practitioner to patient to enhance the body's natural ability to heal itself through the balancing of energy. Reiki utilises specific techniques for restoring and balancing the natural life force energy within the body. It is a holistic, natural, hands-on energy system that touches all levels: body, mind and spirit.

Reiki is believed to have begun in Tibet several thousand years ago. Seers in the Orient studied energies and developed a system of sounds and symbols for universal healing energies. Various healing systems, which crossed many different cultures, emerged from this single root system.

Treatments are ideally given in a quiet peaceful atmosphere with no distractions. While the patient is lying or sitting comfortably, the practitioner simply rests his or her palms on the patient's body and allows the energy to flow. Trying to direct the energy can actually restrict or block its flow, so it is best for the practitioner to take on a passive observant attitude by just being present. In a sense the energy is pulled through the practitioner by the patient's body and goes where it is needed. Only as much as needed will be channelled, you can't channel too much.

The healing hand workout

Below are five separate stretching routines and one all-over mobilisation one, and suggestions as to which are most applicable are included after most of the workouts. However there is no reason why you can't just do one of the relaxing or stretching workouts by themselves. Just make sure you have had an adequate warm-up before you get going.

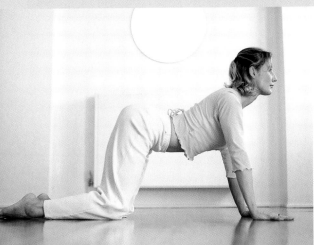

1) BACK AND ABDOMINAL STRETCH

Cat arch

1. Kneeling with your hands on the floor, fingers facing forwards and your hands directly under your shoulders. Knees are in line with your hips. Curve your back downwards to hollow it, at the same time raising your head up.

2. Then slowly arch your back upwards, vertebra by vertebra, into a hunch whilst dropping your head. *Repeat this move slowly about 10 times.*

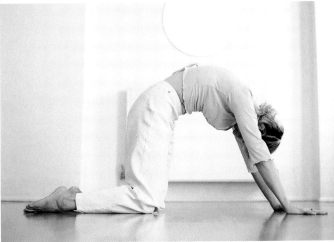

Lower back extensions

1. Lie on the floor on your front, placing your arms out sphinx-like to your sides.

2. Push into your forearms, gently arching through your spine keeping your hips firmly on the floor. Make sure you are not tensing your buttocks or legs. Keep your nose pointing down to the ground and your elbows firmly on the floor. Return slowly to the ground. *Repeat 10 times.*

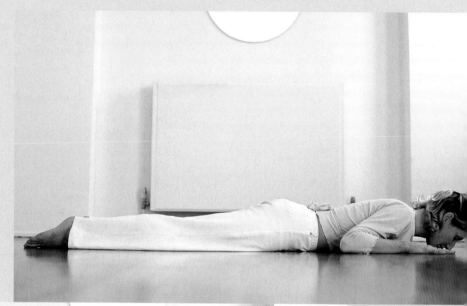

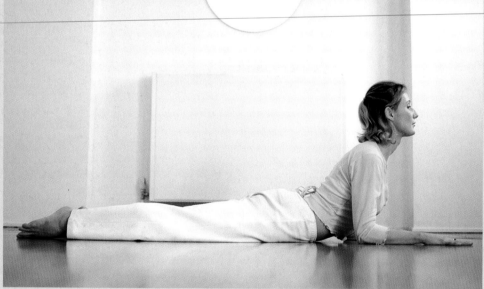

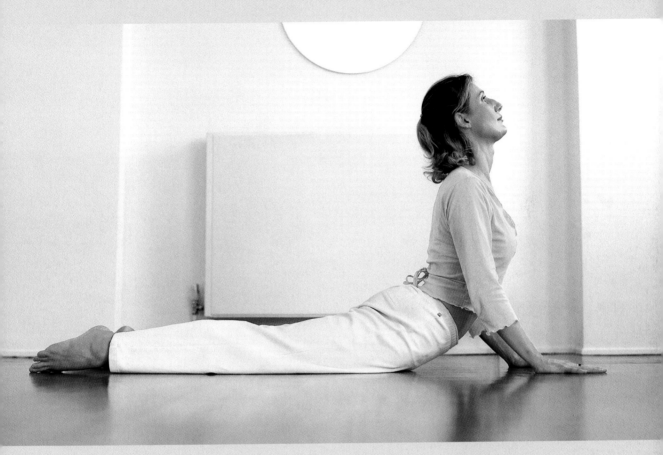

Cobra

Lie on the floor on your stomach, place your hands flat on the floor with your elbows bent and your thumbs level with your armpits. Raise your head up slowly, arching your back. Do not use your arms to push – rather let your back and abdominals do the work. Hold this position for 10 seconds, then try to raise a bit higher for another 10 seconds.

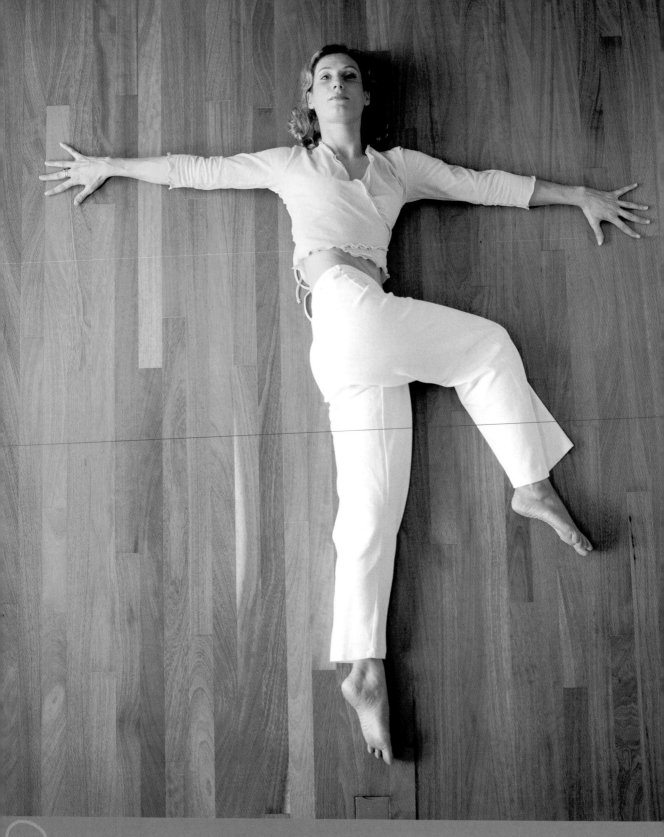

Spinal rotation

<< Lie on your back on the floor with your knees bent and together, and place your feet flat on the floor about hip-width apart. Keeping your shoulders flat on the ground, drop your knees towards the floor to the left. You are aiming to touch your left foot to the right knee without strain. Hold for 20 seconds and repeat other side.

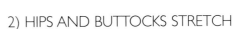

2) HIPS AND BUTTOCKS STRETCH

Inside thigh stretch

Sit on the floor and place your soles of your feet together letting your knees drop open. Hold on to your feet and gently try and press down on your thighs using your elbows. Keep your back straight and your spine long with your chest lifted. Hold for 20 seconds and release.

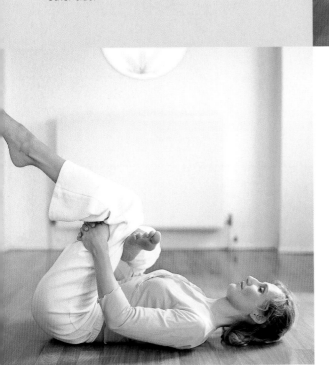

Glute stretch

Lie down on your back with your back flat against the floor and your arms straight by your sides with your palms facing down. Make sure your legs are hip-width apart and the soles of your feet are on the floor. Raise the right leg up towards your upper body and cross it across the left leg. Now bring the left leg upwards so that it is off the floor at almost 90 degrees. At the same time reach through and grasp your left thigh gently drawing both legs towards you. Hold for 20–30 seconds and release. Change sides.

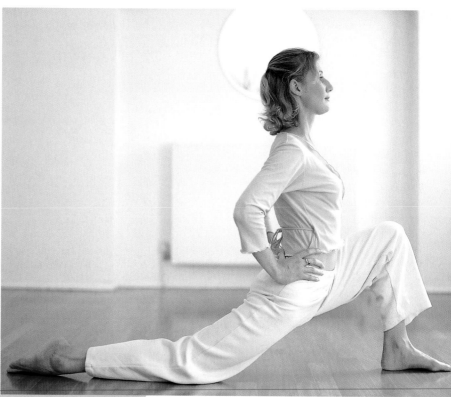

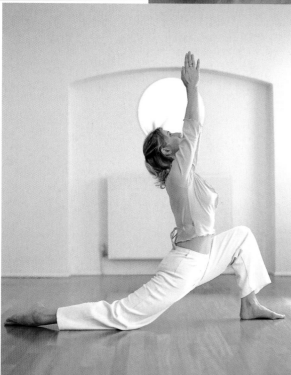

<<

Hip flexors

1. Begin on your knees and then bring your right leg forwards into a right angle. Keep your abdominals tight and body lifted.

2. Gently press your right leg forwards taking care not to let the knee go over the line of the toe. Push the hips forwards looking to feel the stretch in the left hip flexor (front of hip and thigh). Hold for 20 seconds and then release. Change sides.

3) LEGS AND KNEES STRETCH

Dying swan >>

1. Resting on the floor on your hands and knees, extend your left leg straight out behind you.

2. Let your body follow naturally until your chest is resting on your right thigh. Keeping your head and neck relaxed, stay in this position for a few moments. Now begin to use your arms to raise and lower your upper body keeping your legs as they are. Repeat 10 times and then change sides.

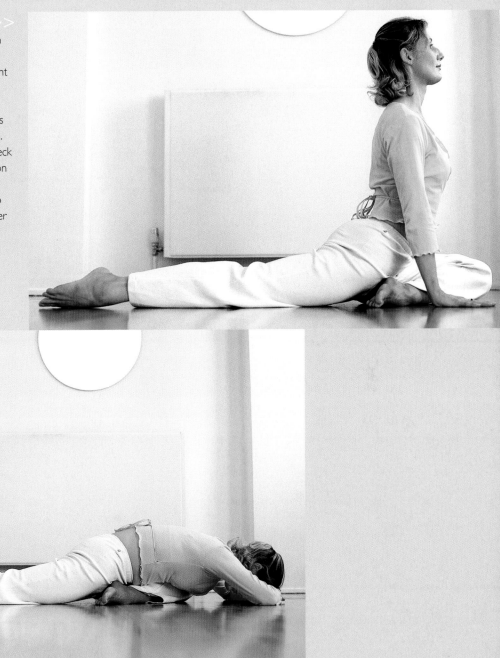

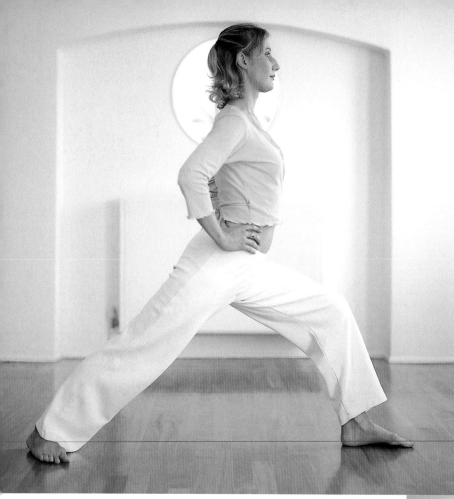

Standing calves

1. Start by standing with your feet hip-width apart. Take your right leg back whilst bending the front knee, pressing your right heel into the ground. Keep your hips and shoulders square and ensure your feet stay hip-width apart for stability. You should feel this stretch in the upper part of the back calf. Hold for 20 seconds and then change legs.

2. For a more advanced stretch, raise your hands above your head as you take your right leg back.

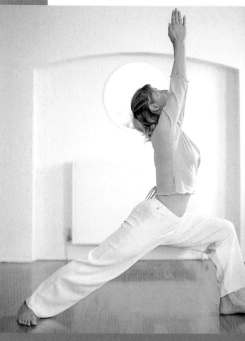

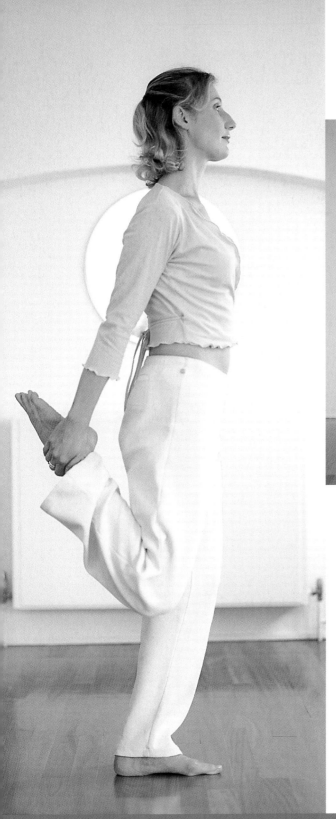

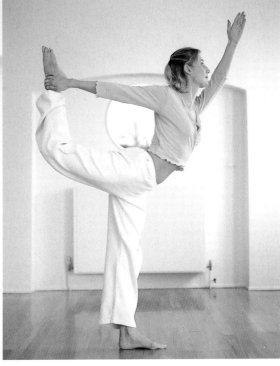

<<

Standing quadriceps

1. Stand with your feet hip-width apart. Reach down with your right hand and gently grasp your right ankle. Draw the heel towards the buttock. Keep the supporting knee soft and your knees parallel. You should feel this stretch along the front of the bent thigh. If you wish to increase this stretch, gently push the hips forwards keeping the knees in line with each other. Hold for 20 seconds and then change sides.

2. For a more advanced stretch, extend the leg further behind you, still holding on to your ankle, and stretch the alternate arm out in front of you for balance.

Downward dog

1. Stand with your feet parallel and hip-width apart, bend over and put your hands flat on the floor about 3 feet in front of you. Push back with your arms, working to get your heels flat on the ground and your head towards the floor. Relax your head and neck letting them hang free.

>>

You should feel a deep stretch along the back of your body. This is a strong and quite difficult stretch and it might take you a while to achieve it.

2. For a more advanced stretch, raise one leg behind you once you are in the above position.

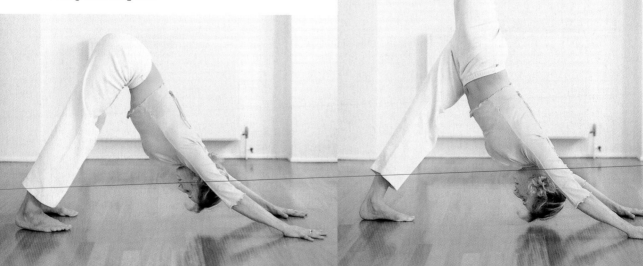

Hip abductors >>

1. Stand in a deep squat position with toes out. Make sure your bottom is not lower than the knees and that your knees go in line with your toes. Place your hands on your thighs gently pressing the legs out. Keep your abdominals tight and your back straight. Hold for 20 seconds.

2. For a more advanced stretch, pivot on one foot whilst stretching the arms straight out at shoulder level.

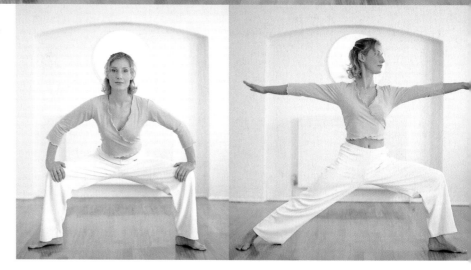

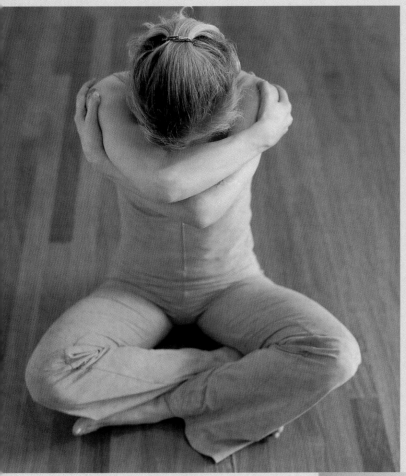

<<

Rhomboid and thoracic

Sit on a chair or a bench, gripping both arms across your chest placing your arms on your shoulders. Now flex your trunk at the upper back as though you are rounding your shoulders and giving yourself a hug. Hold for 20 seconds.

Anterior chest >>

Standing side-on to a wall, place your right hand on the wall at shoulder height. Keeping your right arm straight, turn your feet to the left and rotate your body to left, feeling the stretch across the front of your shoulder. Hold for 20 seconds and then change sides.

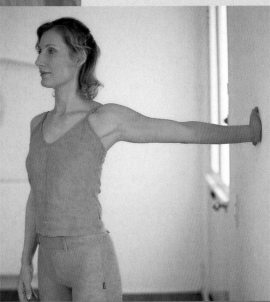

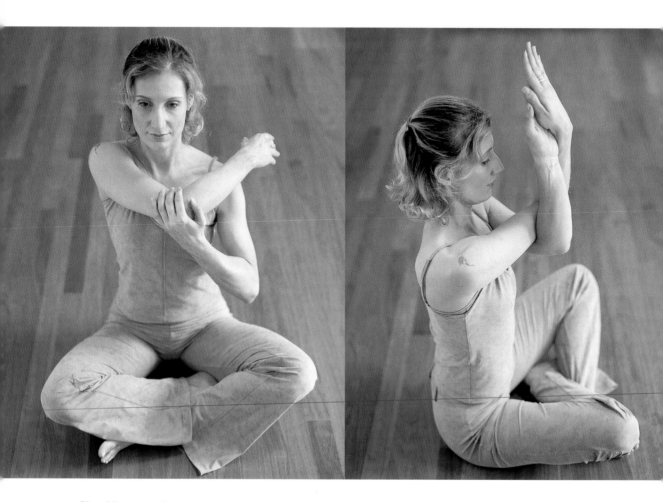

Shoulder stretch

1. Swing your left arm across the front of your body and hook it in with the right forearm. Now gently draw the left arm across looking for a stretch in the back of the left shoulder.

Hold for 20 seconds and then change sides.

2. For a more advanced stretch, cross your arms at the elbow in front of you, with your palms together.

Triceps >>

Stretch the left hand up and drop the palm down between your shoulder blades. Now with the right hand gently push the left upper arm back and slightly down. Hold in this position for 20 seconds and then change sides.

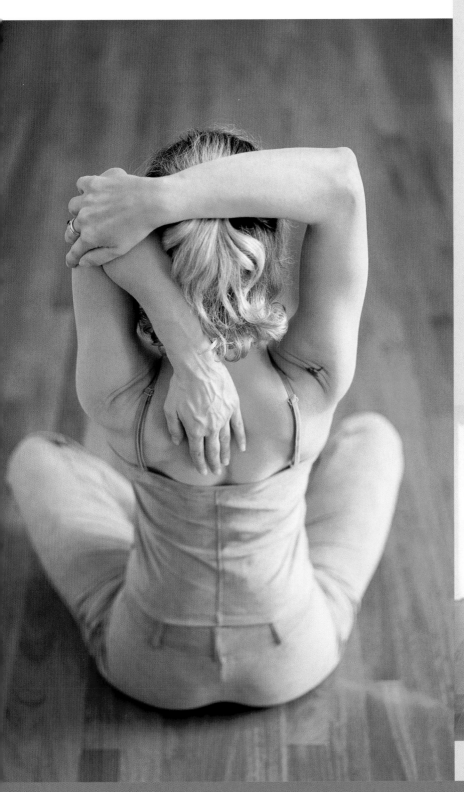

Tower

Sitting with your back straight, interlock your fingers and, with your palms facing up, stretch your arms above your head. Make sure your elbows are straight and your upper arms pulled as far behind your ears as possible. Relax into the move and breathe. Hold for about a minute before resting and repeating. Release your fingers and clasp again with the other thumb on top before repeating.

∨

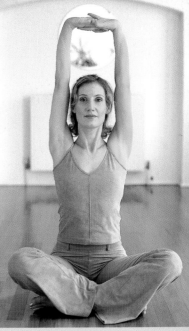

5) QUICK ALL-OVER STRETCH

Lying quads >>

Lie on your front on the floor. Reach down with your right hand and draw your right heel towards your buttock (if you have problems reaching, then wrap a towel or scarf around your ankle and use that to draw the foot up). Keep your hips gently on the floor and your knees hip-width apart. Aim to feel the stretch along the front of the bent thigh. Hold for 20 seconds and then change legs.

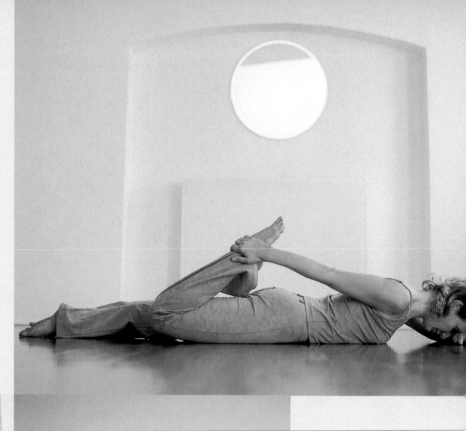

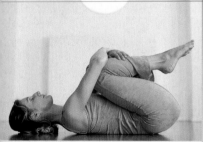

Lower back ball

On your back, draw your knees in towards your chest hugging them with your arms crossed. Make sure your head and neck are relaxed on to the floor. Gently rock from side to side, massaging your spine into the floor. Hold for 20 seconds aiming to stretch out your lower back.

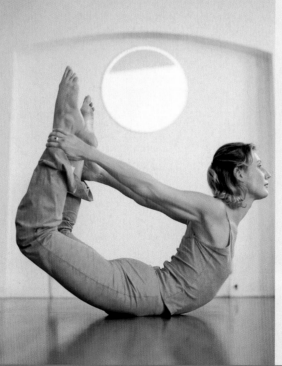

<<

Lying quads

For a more advanced stretch, roll over on to your stomach and clasp your ankles, keeping your head up and looking straight in front of you.

Hamstrings sitting

Sit with your left leg straight and your right leg tucked comfortably in. Sitting up tall, bend forwards from the hips over the straight leg. Try to keep the left foot gently flexed and the base of the knee relaxed into the ground. Come as far forwards as feels comfortable for you and hold. Try and keep your back as straight as possible. Hold for 20 seconds and then change sides.

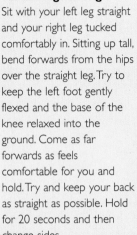

Back and side stretch

Kneeling, place your right hand on your lower hip and stretch up tall with your left hand. Now take your left arm over your head taking your body weight on to the right supporting hand. Hold for 20 seconds and then change sides.

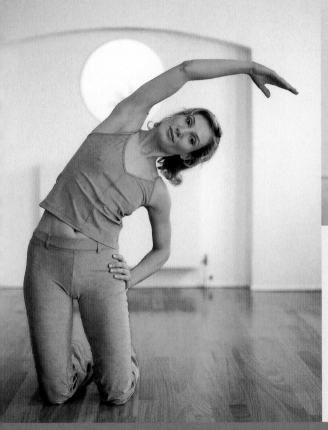

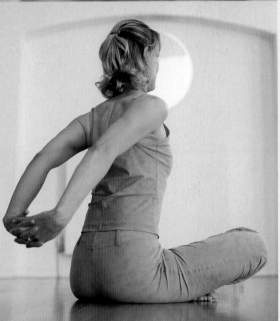

Seated chest stretch

Sit with your back straight. Clasp your hands behind your back and, keeping your elbows slightly bent, draw the hands away from your back. As you do this your shoulders will round back and you will feel your chest 'open'. Hold for 20 seconds and then relax.

Re-energising jumps
This is a great way to finish off any stretch workout. Jump gently and lightly up in the air a few times to release any final tensions. Smile!

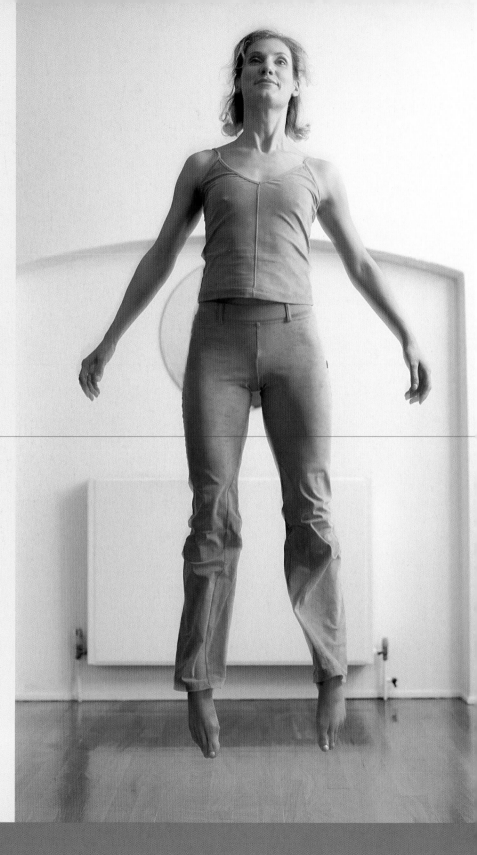

6) FUSION FLEXING

This is a really simple mobilisation routine designed for anyone from six to sixty years old. Use it on its own if you are feeling stiff and lethargic, or add it to your warm-up for an extra special workout.

Upward stretch

Begin with your feet together and your arms at your side. Take a step forwards with your left foot and stretch both arms upwards and forwards. Return to the starting position and repeat with the right leg. Do this 20 times keeping the move smooth and fluid.

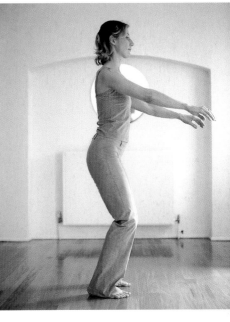

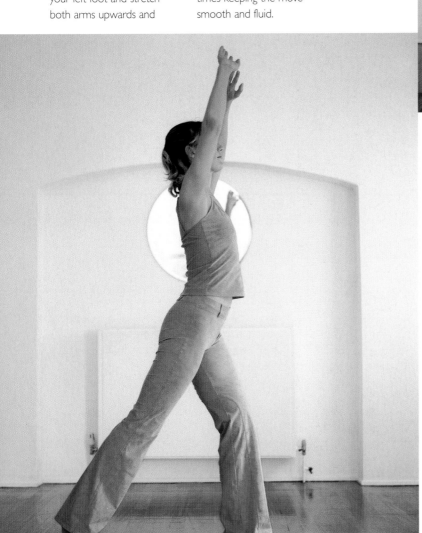

Swinging arms

Start with your feet hip-width apart, knees soft and pelvis tucked under. Your body should be straight, head erect but relaxed and shoulders back and down. Keep your mouth closed with the tip of the tongue placed against the hard palate, eyes looking forwards. Swing both arms forwards and upwards as high as your navel. Then swing downwards and backwards letting them follow through the natural flow. With the swinging of both arms, the lumbar region and pelvis sway forwards and backwards with the same rhythm. Keep your knees soft throughout. Continue for 1–2 minutes. Keep the swinging motion light and effortless, and remember to keep breathing.

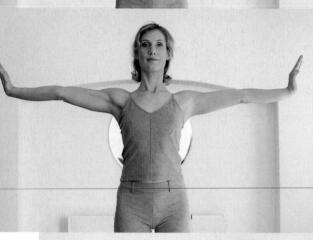

 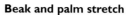

Beak and palm stretch

1. Stand with your feet hip-width apart, knees soft and pelvis tucked naturally under. Lift up your arms to shoulder height whilst clasping your thumb into your tightened inward pointing fingers (as though you are making a 'beak'). Now press out through your wrists feeling a stretch across the top of your wrist and along your arms. Hold for 5–10 seconds.

2. Now draw the hands up whilst bending the elbows and then press out again, this time through the heel of your palm. Hold again for 5–10 seconds.

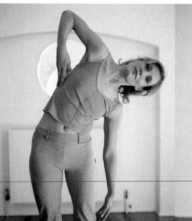 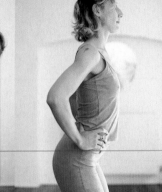

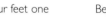

Side bends

Stand with your feet one and a half times hip-width apart, your knees soft and the pelvis tucked naturally under. Place your hands along your sides, keeping the shoulders broad and relaxed. Now stretch down to the right side, taking care to keep the weight even through both feet, Lean neither forwards or back. Return to the centre and repeat other way. Do 10–20 repetitions keeping the move soft and fluid.

Pelvic tilts

Begin with your feet hip width apart, knees soft and your body upright and relaxed. Gently tilt your pelvis forwards tucking your bottom under. Return to the start position taking care not to stick your bottom out behind. Do 10 tilts.

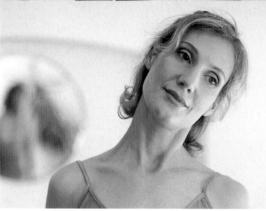

Neck stretch

Stand with your shoulders relaxed and your chest lifted out of your rib-cage. Drop your right ear towards your right shoulder. Keep the shoulders still, relaxed and down during the whole movement. Hold for 5–10 seconds then change sides.

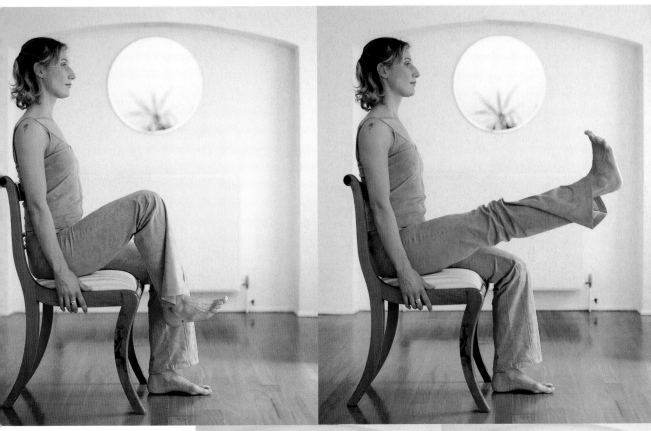

Seated knee extensions

1. Sit in a comfortable straight-backed chair with your feet flat on the floor. Draw your right leg up and in, and then extend it away from you.

2. Press away through the heel but do not lock the knee joint out. Repeat 10 times on each leg keeping the foot gently flexed throughout.

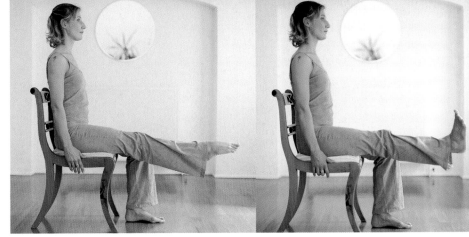

Flexing the feet

1. From the same position as above, raise your right leg out in front of you.

2. Point and flex your foot 10 times before lowering it gently to the ground. Change legs and repeat.

Contacts
The Next Step

Hopefully this book has inspired you to delve further into the world of martial arts. With such a wide range available we have only touched on the surface of international martial art training, so a little investigation into what is available in your area is worthwhile. Umbrella organisations are good starting points.

UK

General Martial Arts

Amateur Martial Assciation (AMA)
66 Chaddesden Lane
Chaddesden
Derby DE21 6LP
Tel: 01332 663086 or 07973 507716

British Council of Chinese Martial Arts
c/o 110 Frensham Drive
Stockingford
Nuneaton
Warwickshire CV10
Tel: 01203 394642

For more information on my company and the individual martial arts teachers and personal trainers we represent:
Fusion Fitness
99 Middle Lane
London N8 8NX
Tel: 020 8374 6087
E-mail: Anne-Marie@Fusionfit.com

The Martial Arts Foundation
PO Box 18253
London EC1N 8FY
E-mail: contact@martialartsfoundation.org
Website: www.martialartsfoundation.org

Jeet Kune Do

Bob Breen's Academy
Hoxton Square
London N1
Tel: 020 7729 5789

Karate

English Karate Governing Body
58 Bloomfield Drive
Bath
Avon BA2 2BG
Tel: 01225 834008

Martin Thompson
martint64@hotmail.com
Personal Fitness Trainer and Holistic Masseur/Sports Therapist who has been practising karate for 20 years.

Kung Fu

British Kung Fu Association
E-mail www.laugar-kungfu.co.uk

Pentjak Silat

Ilan Young
ilanyoung@hotmail.com
Personal Fitness Trainer and Silat Instructor.

Tae Kwon Do

British Tae Kwon Do Council
Otterfield Road
Yiewsley
Middlesex UB7 8PE
Tel: 01895 420722
Fax: 01895 420822

Master Martin Ace
The Martin Ace Black Belt Academy
77 Chichester Road
Edmonton
London N9 9DH
Tel: 020 8345 5128
Website: www.aceman.co.uk
E-mail tkd@aceman.co.uk
Classes and one-to-one lessons.

Tai Chi and Chi Kung

Adam Ali & Ming Ai (London) Institute
Denver House
Cline Road,
London N11 2NG
Tel: 020 8361 7161
Lessons at all levels and Chinese Studies within North London.

Yoga

Becky Mallinson
Tel: 020 8374 3103
Yoga classes and one-to-one personal training in the London area.

AUSTRALIA

General Martial Arts

Australian Martial Arts Association Inc.
PO Box 1272
McLarewn Flat
SA 5171

Silat

Silat Persiai Diri Australia
Tel: 402 305 737

Ju Jitsu

Australian Ju Jitsu Association
Tel: 7 3382 0204

CANADA

Karate

Canadian Shito-Ryu Karate
608 Bellamy Road North
Toronto
Ontario MIH IG7
Tel: 416 708 9258
Website: www.shiotryo.org

Kickboxing

Jean Yves Theriault
Via Instructors Dojo
259 Ste-Anne Street
Vanier
Ontario KIL 7L3
Tel: 613 746 5402

Jean Frenette
1189 du Perche
Boucherville
Quebec J4B 6V3
Tel: 450 641 2775

Tae Kwon Do

Korean Martial Arts Center
126 - B Ontario Aveneue
Elliot Lake
Ontario P5A IY2
Tel: 705 848 3544

NEW ZEALAND

Karate

Australian Toyakwai Karate Association
National Headquarters
Private box 72-1159
Papakura
Auckland
Tel: 9 399 9963

Tae Kwon Do

New Zealand TKD Federation
New Zealand Headquarters
PO Box 14-540
Panmure
Auckland
Tel: 9 570 9228

Wing Chun Kung Fu

Sifu Cheng
P.O. Box 128119
Remuera
Auckland
Tel: 9 571 5403
Website: www.wing-chun.co.nz

Index

AUTHOR ACKNOWLEDGEMENTS

Master Martin Ace
A good friend and one of the best 'teachers' I have come across. Many thanks for all your help, not just with the book, but across the board!

Becky Mallinson
Thank you for making the 'Core Chapter' look so elegant and effortless and for all your expertise in not just the Yoga field but in health and fitness too.

Ilan Young and Martin Thompson
Two of my original Personal Trainers I began working with when I first set up Fusion Fitness (Fighting Fit, as it then was called). Thanks to both of them for all their professional loyalty over the years and their time and effort in helping me with this book.

Adam Ali & Ming Ai (London) Institute
Best wishes and thanks to both of the above. Especially thanks to Adam for his help and knowledge of Tai Chi and Chi Kung, not just within this book but for all the other times I have called upon him.

Finally with thanks to **Savash Mustafa**, for being the best Osteopath, patiently looking after myself and my clients and for answering the many queries that I throw at him!

The publisher would also like to thank Casalls (c/o Viva (UK) Limited, 2 Market Place, Somerton, Somerset, TA11 7LX; 01458 273394) for kindly loaning sports clothes for the photoshoots.